# Fighting Back

# Fighting Back

## One Woman's Struggle Against Cancer

*Joie Harrison McGrail*

**HARPER & ROW, PUBLISHERS**

New York, Hagerstown, San Francisco, London

FIGHTING BACK: ONE WOMAN'S STRUGGLE AGAINST CANCER. Copyright © 1978 by the Estate of Joie Harrison McGrail. All rights reserved. Printed in the United States of America. No part of this book may be used or reproduced in any manner whatsoever without written permission except in the case of brief quotations embodied in critical articles and reviews. For information address Harper & Row, Publishers, Inc., 10 East 53rd Street, New York, N.Y. 10022. Published simultaneously in Canada by Fitzhenry & Whiteside Limited, Toronto.

FIRST EDITION

Designed by Stephanie Krasnow

Library of Congress Cataloging in Publication Data

McGrail, Joie.
    Fighting back.
    1. Lungs—Cancer—Biography.   2.   McGrail, Joie.
I.   Title.
RC280.L8M23 1978        362.1'9'699424        76-26244
ISBN 0-06-012958-1

78  79  80  10  9  8  7  6  5  4  3  2  1

My thanks to my son, Richard Harrison, who edited my manuscript,
and to Phyllis Nevins, creative associate.

# Contents

# Fighting Back

# CHAPTER I

# On a Perfect Day in June

A small, iridescent rainbow danced down my face, and my laugh of delight cut through the warm mist. I wrapped myself twice around with an oversized Turkish towel and stepped into the patch of sunshine that flooded in through the bathroom skylight. The apothecary jars broke the rays into little spectra, and the mound of pink towels reflected a rosy glow through the room.

My cheeks glowed rosy, too, in the still-fogged mirror. As the fog cleared off, I faced the glass squarely, happy that at fifty-two I still was pleased by the image looking back.

I rummaged through the jars and bottles to find an old, seldom-used lilac perfume. The sentimental fragrance enveloped me, evoking sympathetic vibrations of all the lilacs locked within me from all of the summers of my life.

I was still humming the refrain of a long-ago song as I breezed into the kitchen, and our happy herd of cats joined me in a purr chorus as they rubbed around the hem of my kimono, waiting for breakfast. Bill had risen earlier, so a big glass of fresh orange juice and a pot of coffee were waiting on a wicker table that had been set up to catch the first bit of sunlight that filtered through the trees to the patio. I was very glad we had decided to stay in the country for the week, even though it would mean an eighty-mile drive to the airport later in the morning.

It was going to be hard to tear myself away from this perfect day with Bill, but an important project of mine was finally about to be realized and the trip was really necessary. One meeting was with a U.S. Department of State official, the other with a Latin American diplomat. Neither could possibly be canceled.

I went out to the little table in the sun as soon as the cats had settled into their buffet. Bill stopped his gardening and came over to join me with an armful of just-cut roses for the crock on the table. "You smell different today; did you run out of your regular perfume?" How he could tell, over the glorious scent of that armful of roses, was beyond me. "No, I just felt sentimental today."

Once the roses were arranged in the crock Bill gave them a hearty drink from a watering pail. We turned to our breakfast and devoured a tray of fresh buttermilk biscuits drenched in home-made strawberry preserves.

Two important meetings awaited, but now the only important thing was the after-breakfast walk with Bill in our sun-sparkled garden. Our patio breakfasts always end with a ritual "tour of the grounds," a casual meander through the masses of plants that crowd every inch of our country place and turn it into a gigantic flowerpot. Snippets of night-blooming jasmine, smuggled back from a visit to Morocco, now tower over the roof. Bougainvillea from our honeymoon on the Italian Riviera mingles with its Puerto Rican cousin; giant Brazilian amaryllis grow as lushly in earthen urns as in their awesome natural habitat. Our plants are our passion and our souvenirs—a living joy and remembrance of pleasures past.

That day the woods were a cathedral of beautiful forms and fragrances. I worshipped in in my fashion, remembering the young times when I skipped church to stand alone in a grove of mountain laurel. As the light streamed between the trees, I drew closer in silent communion with my husband. We were so fortunate, Bill and I . . . a second marriage for both of us, a happy merging of families; his two sons and two daughters, my grown son, all living in different parts of the world now, but all close in thought and love. Bill and I were fortunate too, to have each other and savor our lives as passionate participants in such a wide range of interests: we loved to collect antiques, *objets d'art*, old stuff, junk; we loved to travel; we loved to fish for trout complete with all of the traditional refinements of fragile fly rods and hand-tied flies or to go after big bluefish rough-house, with chunky boat rods on our Jersey skiff. Our passion approached mania for horticulture, cats, and good cuisine. We were always together in essential bond, even when the demands of our busy careers sometimes sent us in different directions. Separation was only a prelude to reunion and today's separation would be only a short one . . . I'd be flying home on the evening shuttle, anxious not to lose an hour of our country time.

I am not normally a clock watcher, but I do plan my day in advance and some finely tuned reflex moves me from one thing to another at the appointed time. But on this beautiful June morning I had gotten so lost in reverie there amid the mountain laurel, honeysuckle and a perfumed patch of lilac, that I had lost track of time. I hurriedly kissed Bill goodbye, for by the time I would be dressed and ready to be off, he'd be lost somewhere among the plants. As I darted toward the house, Bill called:

"How about dinner in the gazebo tonight?"

"It's a date!"

Although I've flown often and far as business and pleasure have taken me around the world, a lingering tendency to landing sickness still embarrasses me occasionally. Today the Washington shuttle was nearly empty so I had two seats to myself, and I immediately filled the second one with stacks of yellow paper as I worked on the last-minute insights that seem to sharpen well-developed ideas. The flight was so smooth that I just worked on, hardly noticing the pilot's announcement that we'd be landing shortly. There was no tedious circling, only the beginning of a gliding descent . . . and absolutely no reason whatsoever for the shocking wave of nausea that flooded me. I bent double, hoping I wouldn't be sick. The nausea mounted . . . and then pain stabbed the left side of my chest, stabbed and stabbed again until I gasped out ragged breath. I still clutched a piece of paper in my left hand, and I couldn't open my fingers again. I could feel a heavy, throbbing pain in my left arm that made me groan, but I couldn't make it work, not a finger, not a muscle. It hurt terribly and seemed paralyzed. I thought, My God, what a case of landing sickness. How embarrassing. I hope no one has noticed! I suffered through locked teeth, concentrating on the moment when the plane's wheels would touch the ground; we'd roll, we'd stop . . . and all this would disappear. I held that thought while we touched down, rolled to a stop . . . but the pain got worse. Now it was a monstrous squeezing, the closing and closing of a fist around my heart. I was sticky, I was drenched, soaking, shower-wet, gushing sweat as if the fist were wringing me dry from the inside out. I didn't move because I couldn't, and finally a stewardess came to me.

"Do you need any help?"

"No, thank you," I managed to answer.

No, because it was airsickness and it would pass. I waited as the other passengers filed out of the plane. Still I sat, and she came again. Was I ill? I hardly heard her. This couldn't be illness, illness had nothing to do with me, I had never been ill in my life. I told myself with the same exquisite sequence of logic that since this was the case, and since I wasn't really ill, I must make myself move and get off this plane. I sent out orders to my legs and working arm. Move! Lift the dead weight and support it on the briefcase! Get up! Walk! My body has never failed me and I didn't think of failure now. I thought, Left, right, left, right . . . I began to shuffle forward. It was motion of a sort; it got me to the cabin door. The waiting stewardess insisted: "Please, won't you let me help you?" It was difficult to answer her, difficult to break my concentration of will, but I raised my chin with the stiff pride of a drunk defending his sobriety. "No, thank you. I'm fine."

Fine! I don't know what she thought of my sweat-drenched face, hunched arm, wooden walk, but it didn't matter because I did not need to ask her for help, and I stumbled past her out of the plane, down the ramp and into the terminal.

There was no question of stopping. I didn't dare stop. Forward, keep moving forward. My left arm was still supported on the right that held the briefcase, but I had to drag my body forward each time I put a foot down, and each time I did, my head lurched and I could imagine my picture-hat's large brim quivering and fluttering like a desperate bird. A corner of my mind not concerned with the effort of moving forward marveled at the absurdity. People near me reacted with staring concern. They'd start forward to offer help, but when their eyes met mine, my grim determination discouraged any further thought of meddling. Did they whisper, "Drunk?" "Drugged?" "What's wrong with her?" It didn't matter. I was making it alone, with the vise in my chest screwed tight, and my determination to go on alone dispersed the staring Samaritans. Only one trailed me. A nice-looking young man followed at a discreet distance and when I finally blundered against a bench and went down stiffly, he was standing at a nearby newsstand, waiting.

Reaching the bench reaffirmed my confidence. I had made it this far and that meant I could continue. I had proved my unassailability and now the worst was over—it would surely pass, this damned, horrible, humiliating nuisance of a pain would leave me. I looked up. The young man was waiting for some slight signal that his intervention would be welcomed and I tried to reassure him wordlessly. I gazed back with what I thought of as élan, hat askew and sweat still trickling down my face. I tried for a gracious nod, an "I'm all right, thank you" nod, but my version of it brought him over instantly.

"You look ill. Can I help?"

It wasn't embarrassing after all; his directness made me suddenly grateful.

"I don't know quite what happened. It started when the plane was landing and I thought it was extreme airsickness, but the pain in my chest and arm . . . and this perspiration . . ."

"I think I'd better get you to a hospital. I believe you've had a heart attack."

"Heart attack? That's impossible!" But he certainly meant well and he could be of help if he wanted to bring me a glass of buttermilk. "Buttermilk?" It was his turn to be flabbergasted.

I explained that I'd often had buttermilk in the coffee shop while waiting for a return flight to New York. Buttermilk is my own private wonder drug.

He humored me and brought it, watching while I drank it slowly.

Slow swallows. Slowed speech. Everything moving at a fraction of its usual speed, but at least my voice was clear and I could concentrate.

He asked me what I meant to do next. I already knew. I'd rent a private bath stall in the ladies' room of a downtown hotel, a haven where I'd often repaired accidents of travel. I smiled, telling him that I deprecated the soggy Washington climate that usually made such repairs necessary. It was normal conversation, I think, because I was breathing more easily and concentrating my will on exorcising the pain. When I did stand up, it was manageable! Small, measured steps on my Galahad's arm brought me to a taxi stand. He wouldn't leave me; he helped me in and rode with me to the hotel.

I think my kind, nameless young man saw some visible improvement in me on the ride downtown. I'd regained a little of the light touch, enough so that when we said goodbye, my friend had lost his look of tragic anxiety and while he admonished me to see a doctor and ''be careful,'' he didn't repeat his suggestion that he get me to a hospital.

We said goodbye. Of course I would be careful. But I was so much more myself after a bit of rest, some buttermilk and sympathy, that I could tell the alarmed matron in the ladies' room, who had earlier known a much less disheveled me, that it was all the result of a very rough trip. I sent her for the biggest Turkish towel available and stepped into a cubicle complete with shower and cot.

I finally looked in a mirror. An attractive woman in an elegant hat had gotten on the plane this morning . . . Medusa looked back at me now.

But rest, renewal, and what was in my makeup kit would fix all that. I tried to settle down on the cot. One position was the most bearable, but any quick motion brought back the excruciating squeeze on my heart. And the left arm—it still lay there. But there was time: it was only 10:15 and my appointment wasn't until noon.

I realize now that my priorities were lunatic! Rest and cosmetic repair, keeping a luncheon appointment. This, while pain still hovered, arm still dragged, and life might be running out in minutes of delay, if, as I'd been told, I'd just walked through a heart attack. But I was incapable of comprehending illness in myself. I had no reference point for incapacitating illness. In my entire life, I'd never suffered a sickness and my consciousness of even passing, momentary pain had been so minimal that I'd never taken an aspirin. The only times I'd seen a doctor since I broke my leg while skiing twenty years before was when I needed shots for my International Health card when I was traveling off the beaten path. I'd always accepted and enjoyed my health and stamina as a state of grace, a natural consequence of instinctive adherence to nature's laws. I had never used hard alcohol or cigarettes. My reverence for nature was not a whim: I was in balance with the natural world around me, and that balance was a source of deep contentment. As a child I'd spurned the bathtub in the family summer cottage for a ritual icy morning dip at a mountain spring. For pleasure, I've swum in lakes at dawn; ridden horseback over trails that others avoided. The grass was greener for me, the flowers more fragrant, because I knew the natural world and was part of it—not just a spectator. Perfect balance had brought me perfect health, and if it momentarily slipped, the balance would right itself as it always had. Although I was shocked and frightened by the sudden, strange attack, I didn't see it as the possible end of my charmed existence.

Each action of renewal, awkward as it was, reasserted my sense of invulnerable self. I undressed—not easily—and hung my silk suit to steam out wrinkles in the shower's warm vapors. I wrapped my ruined hair in towels, cleaned my face with astringent, and when the vapor filling the air made it easier to breathe, I dropped into a deep sleep.

My silence and the non-stop running water must have frightened the matron outside. Her knocking woke me. I moved cautiously to turn off the shower and open the door a crack.

"Are you sure you're all right? Is there anything I can do?"

I sent her for a glass of buttermilk.

She brought it and also a hair dryer for my damp, scraggly hair. The restoration moved along slowly because the simplest action called for complicated logistics: how to shower and towel without moving your body, how to maneuver that dead arm into a sleeve, how to pull a buttonhole over a button. But the time came when I had recreated my face and even replaced the hat with the quivering brim. There was one forlorn moment when a touch of perfume brought back the morning's extravagance of lilac . . . how far away that happiness seemed now.

It was time to plan for the exigencies of my day. Luncheon with the Ambassador would include the ritual of handshaking. Fortunately, the useless hand was my left and not the right. And there would be problems with chairs, with the knife and fork. Still, I could make the best of it, keep pleasant and presentable, carry it through. And the other appointment, the State Department conference, was fully three hours away. In three hours I might well be back to normal. Even now I found that if I stood erect and just slightly inclined to the left from the waist up, I could handle the pain. Yes, a little discipline would do it.

His Excellency began to show me to a deep, soft armchair, which would turn into a trap. I asked whether I couldn't have the pleasure of using a magnificent carved antique instead, thinking that the higher seat, straight back and firm arms would give me more support. I settled into it fairly easily, and once seated, noted with relief that the pain seemed to have subsided almost completely. My left hand looked natural enough resting lightly in my lap, and I found that I could even move around a bit.

Once the discussion got under way, my discomfort receded. We had a lot to talk about. I had been commissioned by an affluent Midwestern corporation to coordinate a Latin American exposition for the following summer. The arts, the handicrafts, the fashions, the foods and the principal products of the area would be transported to the Midwest for a month-long gala. A year's work lay behind me and a year's work still lay ahead. I became so engrossed that I forgot my physical condition completely and enjoyed the animated and successful meeting, without any reminder of my weird attack.

When the butler came in to announce lunch, however, I realized that I would have to try to manage a very formal meal one-handed. I never did get to the solution of that problem, for as we rose to go to the dining room, the vise was turning in my chest again and my left arm felt as if it were being mangled. With as little drama as possible I said, "Your Excellency, excuse me, but I'm afraid that I am ill." I asked that he call my friends at the State Department to ask them to arrange for me to be taken to a hospital.

It seemed strange to hear myself saying "hospital," for the notion of being sick was still beyond my comprehension. I didn't have long to think about the strangeness, however, for I was the center of a flurry of concern and activity. The Ambassador wanted to call a doctor immediately but before he did, an aide had Sam Belk at the State Department on the phone. He said that he would be right there to take me to the Georgetown University Hospital while an associate called to alert the hospital and a cardiologist that I was coming.

Three hours later, instead of being in conference, I was tête-à-tête with an electrocardiogram machine that twitched pulses from my body and recorded my heart's activity on graph paper. With the help of my friend Sam I had been admitted to the Emergency Room, and I was in fragments. My possessions had disappeared into hospital safekeeping, my elegant white silk suit slung on a hook in a locker, my hat (too big for the locker) had been taken by Sam to his State Department office, and my heart and mind were reaching out to Bill in New York. He didn't know!

The doctors knew something, but didn't tell me. They asked questions, but answered none of mine. What was going to happen? A cardiac specialist would see me. They would keep me overnight. They might put me in Intensive Care. Unreal, eerie, but it was happening. Worse, there was an irresistible sense of process, of being drawn into a system and subject to its rules. I was out of my own control now. For the first time in my life.

# CHAPTER II

# The Doughnut on
# the X-ray

GEORGETOWN UNIVERSITY HOSPITAL

McGRAIL, JOIE

HISTORY OF PRESENT ILLNESS: This fifty-two-year-old white female, appearing younger than her stated age, was admitted on 6/20/74 to the Coronary Care Unit because of a three-hour history of a substernal chest pain radiating to the left arm.

HOSPITAL COURSE: In the CCU serial EKGs and enzymes were not indicative of acute myocardial injury; however EKG revealed the presence of old Q waves in leads I, III and AVF. This was compatible with old anterior wall myocardial infarction.

This entry from the hospital log indicates that something had happened to my heart before. But when? I had never had a heart attack. Yet the machine had given me a history, consigned me to the Coronary Care Unit, and there I lay, strapped down against unnecessary movement, wired in to the monitor recording my heart action and sporting an intravenous feeding needle in the large vein of my taped-to-a-board left hand. Around me was a silent circle of what I thought of as the real cardiac cases: gray-faced, inert, some beyond caring, though well cared for by a large number of cheerful nurses. But if the others were motionless, I itched to move! Feeling prickled into the fingers of my left hand, the chest pain was episodic, receding. I tried to tell the nurses that I was feeling better, but they hushed me maternally—no exertion, please. CCU was as quiet as a sleeping nursery with all its occupants cocooned in white sheets and wired in to the mother-monitor.

One of the alert, energetic young nurses who were bustling back and forth between patients and machines came over to my bed. "Hi, I'm Anna." She chirped that my color was good, and asked me to repeat what had happened.

I had barely begun, when a distinguished, scholarly-looking man approached. I liked the cardiologist at first sight. His slightly stooped posture seemed to radiate a sympathetic gentleness—and the slouch reminded me immediately of my son. "Hello, Mrs. McGrail," he said. "I'm here at the request of your friend Sam Belk. Please tell me exactly what happened. And give me every detail, even those which might seem trivial to you." And so I gave my history once again.

The doctor listened attentively and took notes. He examined me carefully, studied the various graphs made by the machines I had been plugged into, and inspected the record which the nurse gave him. He told me that he had ordered more tests for the following day, and would be able to reach a more specific diagnosis after seeing the results. He gave Anna some instructions, said goodbye and left. It somehow seemed to be too quick. And he hadn't discovered any mistake. He obviously felt that I belonged right there in cardiac intensive care.

I could see that most of my questions would go unanswered in the hospital, where the patient, importunate child, is tucked in, trundled from one place to another, told how sick he is or what he can and can't do, all on the operative principle that "Mommy knows best.'' Hospitals, by their very nature, tend to do your thinking for you. I'd discovered this cottonwool barrier when I'd first tried to telephone Bill from the Emergency Room.

A white-coated young resident had come to tell me that I would be transferred to the Cardiac Intensive Care Unit in a few minutes, and asked where the hospital might phone my husband, since it had to notify him. I was startled. ''I'll speak to my husband myself, if you'll bring me a phone, please,'' I told him. ''You can't do that,'' he said. ''It's against the rules. The hospital has to call him.''

''Why is it against the rules?'' I asked. ''Surely you don't want to promote another cardiac infarction, or whatever you think this is.'' Bill had never seen me sick. I could imagine his shock if a hospital called and said I was in Cardiac Intensive Care. ''Cardiac patients cannot be taxed with telephone conversations,'' the young man answered. ''Besides, you're on your way to Intensive Care, and there are no telephones there.''

''My dear young man, you and your colleagues have just been taxing me at great length to repeat the history of whatever has happened to me over and over. Furthermore, this conversation is more taxing than a telephone call to my husband. I intend to speak to my husband even if it means I've got to unplug myself and walk to the nearest telephone booth.'' He seemed to find some logic in what I'd said, for he good-naturedly handed over a telephone.

I tried the country place without luck. But I had an idea. I was sure that Bill would be checking in with the answering service in the city toward the end of the day. I dialed our city number and got the answering service operator we'd had for years. ''Hello, Mrs. McGrail, I have some messages.'' I interrupted quickly, not sure how long my grace period on the phone would last. ''No, Mary, I don't want any messages now. I want you to listen very carefully and do exactly what I tell you.'' ''Yes, ma'am, is anything wrong?''

"Well, yes, there is. I'm in Georgetown University Hospital. Take that down, write it clearly. It appears that I've had a heart attack. No, no, Mary, please don't fuss . . ." But she had begun to wail "Oh, God!" over and over again.

"Mary, you must listen closely and don't become distracted, or you won't be able to give Mr. McGrail the message the way I want you to give it to him." She was choking back "no's" under her breath, so I gave her a moment to compose herself and then went on. "Now, I wouldn't be talking to you like this if I were about to die, would I? It's not that kind of a heart attack. It's a little one." And though I believed this was true, I said it because I knew I had to convince her, or else her voice would terrify Bill when she gave him the message.

"Make certain that when you talk to Mr. McGrail you tell him that you talked to me personally. Tell him I'm going into the Cardiac Care Unit and that he won't be able to call me, but that I'm not in danger." I knew that Bill would have to drive two hours to the airport, then possibly wait for a flight, fly down, then get to the hospital. It could be four or five hours from the time he got the message until he got to the hospital. I didn't want him to spend those hours wondering whether I was going to be dead or alive upon his arrival.

"Also, Mary, please make certain to ask Mr. McGrail to tell my son that I spoke to you personally." I knew that Bill would call Dick no matter what I said, so I hoped that this would at least minimize the shock. Dick lived abroad and although I found myself thinking how nice it would be to see him, since he hadn't been in New York for months, I was very concerned about interrupting his busy life, and about having him worry until he could get away to Washington.

"Mary really has her work cut out for her," said the young white-coat as I finally relinquished the phone. Then he and two others wheeled me off to Intensive Care.

The nurse bustled from my bedside to the glass booth on an

endless round. Each visit distracted me for just a bit from my confusion and the growing irritation and feeling of indignity over being strapped down and wired in to all that machinery. Finally, on one visit she said that she had just spoken to Bill, who had called on his way to the airport. He would arrive at seven, and Dick and his wife Stephanie would be getting in the next morning. I was happy and relieved, for I did need the support they all would bring.

I've always heard that you can't sleep in hospitals in spite of sleeping pills. I was given none, but the sheer mindless waiting itself was an effective soporific. The world dwindled to the compass of objects closest to my bed. Everything else seemed impossibly far out of reach. The blinking lights of the monitor might be a distant galaxy, the nurses peripheral beings, the other patients blurs of white. Bit by bit, as I focused on a bedside glass of water, the world slipped away. Sheer, mindless, strapped-down, wired-in waiting in the void finally hypnotized me into sleep.

When I woke up Bill was standing at my bedside. He always looked tall beside me, but as I lay there strapped into all of the leather and wire attachments, he seemed to tower over me. And I came to the terrible realization that I had lost my freedom. There was Bill beside me, and I couldn't reach out to him and walk away with him. I was helpless. We both were. This thing had taken over our lives, everything had been shattered, possibly never to be the same again. And then I felt the first cold shudder of fear.

Bill pulled a chair close to my bed and sat down. He looked anxious and shocked, but I scrutinized him carefully and could see that he wasn't terrified. Good. That meant that he too thought that this was a fluke. The doctor had probably just overreacted to my symptoms because I had overreacted. We'd clear it up in the morning. "You look great," said Bill. "Nothing like a heart attack patient. In fact, you don't look any different than you did this morning, and that was pretty snappy.'' He stroked some stray wisps of hair away from my cheek. "But your hairdo was prettier then." He patted my hand, taped to its wooden support, and asked whether it hurt very much. "Not now," I told him, then recited the saga of my day's misadventures.

The barrage of tests and examinations began early the next morning. It seemed that different specialists were coming and going to check every function and part of me. They even wheeled in a portable X-ray machine. Finally the nurse said that there would be an hour's break. I asked whether I could tidy up a bit. It was a treat to perform all of my customary morning rituals. It seemed that the Cardiac Intensive Care Unit had an endless supply of cheerful nurses, for the morning nurse seemed simply delighted to hold a mirror while my right hand went through its familiar paces. Even the left was able to contribute a bit, even though it was plugged into the intravenous feeding tube and strapped to a board. I surveyed the results and was relieved to see that I looked no different than usual.

Now my attention was riveted on the entrance door. Soon a tall, handsome familiar form bolted into the room. "Dick! I'm here, at the end." A few long strides brought him to my bedside, his usually serious face a perfect study in tension. He took a long look at me and smiled. "You look fine." He was visibly relieved, and I was relieved to see that he was smiling. He had my smile, but he didn't wear it as often. He had always teased me about my eternal optimism, and I despaired of his incurable skepticism; so the fact that he looked pleased meant a great deal. If such a determined realist as he didn't appear too worried, things couldn't be all that bad.

I asked for Stephanie, and Dick said that she was setting up housekeeping nearby. A bachelor friend of theirs who occasionally visited with them and had repeatedly invited them to come to stay with him in Washington had had his invitation taken up on short notice. Serendipity! He lived in Georgetown, just a few blocks from the hospital. I was aghast at the inconvenience they must have caused by calling one afternoon and showing up the following morning. "Stephanie felt the same," said Dick. "She thought that Jeff would be up all night sprucing the place up. But he just shoveled the socks out of the living room and let it go at that. Stephanie is spending a couple of hours making our room habitable." Bill joined us then, and after a brief visit they both went off to talk with the doctor, promising to return with Stephanie in the afternoon.

I was sorry to see them go, for everything seemed so much better when they were around. Bill and I had been like newly-weds for fifteen years, and Dick and I had never allowed his independent adulthood to interfere with the fact that we loved each other dearly. It would be nice to look forward to their afternoon visit through the day of tests.

The cardiologist came to continue his examination and we got back down to the business of getting my history. Apparently my recital of yesterday was only the beginning. "Think back," the doctor urged. "Do you recall any episode prior to this, when you might have had similar pains or symptoms?"

"Oh, no" I answered . . . and suddenly remembered the time six weeks earlier, when one of our pet cats had been killed. My snow-white Wynken was the survivor of twins. Blynken, her brother, had died violently a few weeks earlier, and now Wynken was struck by a car in the lane that fronted our country place. I remembered finding her body. She lay silky white with no sign of violent death, except the frozen fear in her amber eyes and a bright blotch of blood, a red gourd that flowed out of her mouth and onto the road. I'd knelt beside Wynken's body and wept deep moans from some unknown inner place. First, Blynken had died of convulsions after being poisoned by a neighbor's chlordane-treated lawn. Now, only two weeks later, Wynken was the victim of a speeding car. My anguish was double and what could I think but that the burning, squeezing sensation that surrounded my heart with fire was a physical manifestation of that anguish? Pain immobilized me then, just as it would weeks later on the plane. I spent most of the weekend of Wynken's death huddled in grief and pain on a couch, knowing that Bill was grieving too while he immersed himself in chores. I remember thinking with a touch of awe, How can my broken heart be so painful physically?

My doctor's expression told me that this thing I had forgotten—or perhaps blocked out—was very important. Apparently I had had some sort of cardiac infarction, or "clogging," at the time of Wynken's death, and then again on the plane.

The doctor was relieved that there had been an event which confirmed his reading of the EKGs. "That does square with the evidence as we see it, but the nature of the disturbance is as yet not identified. Anyway, there is no need for you to stay here any longer; you can move into a private room tomorrow, and we'll have the rest of our tests done in a few days. By then I hope we will be able to identify the source of the mystery. You can resume most normal activities right now." That news lifted my spirits wonderfully. I could get unplugged, eat, walk around—perhaps even take a bath. And it must surely mean that I'd be on my way home in no time.

Stephanie, Dick and Bill were elated. I was impatient to have the tests done and go home. We made a strange group for a family in an Intensive Care Unit. They were gleefully planning a treat for my lunch the next day and asked what I wanted most. "What I really want is one of Stephanie's quiches, but since you're settled in bachelor quarters, I'll settle for a treat from one of the little specialty places in the neighborhood." Dick was wondering whether I'd be permitted a sip of wine, when the doctor returned. His nervous, almost embarrassed attitude stopped us in mid-smile. He started to stammer something about the unreliability of portable X-ray units, then blurted out:

"There seems to be a large density on the lung, a doughnut-shaped shadow appears on the X-ray. I just got the radiologist's report and came right over." It was strange to see him so shaken, when he had been so calm, even on his first visit to me in the Intensive Care Unit. Bill, Dick and Stephanie seemed to have frozen. And then I read in their faces the word the doctor couldn't bring himself to say: *cancer*. But it was impossible. I had never smoked a cigarette in my life. I had avoided chemicals, never took any kind of pill. It couldn't possibly be cancer. The doctor found his composure again. "It's probably a faulty unit. Those portable X-ray machines are notorious. Might also be bad film, but I suspect a faulty unit. In any event, I've ordered a series of X-rays for you tomorrow morning, just after you move into your room."

We were stunned and took a few moments to grapple with the enormity of the potential calamity. Then, simultaneously, as if on some signal, we all began to reassure each other that the doctor had said that the portable units were faulty, or that the film could have been bad. We got back to the subject of the next day's lunch, and decided that a sip of wine was definitely in order. We were all bantering bravely before it was time to leave. After I had kissed my family goodbye and they were out the door, I hoped that I had done a better job than they had in looking cheerful. I then turned to the business at hand: overcoming the fear that seemed ready to creep into any weakness I left open; reminding myself to wait for facts and not to worry in advance—willing out of my mind the catalogue of horrors that the word "cancer" conjured up.

When I awakened the next morning, I was moved out of Intensive Care without delay. My new room had what must be the loveliest view in Georgetown: a gently rolling grassy hillside leading up to a ridge line forested over with tall old trees. There was no house in sight. The only visible residents were some horses grazing in paddocks set apart by rustic split-rail fences. I enjoyed my breakfast, my first food in two days. Then I used my new freedom to luxuriate in a bath. I wrapped myself in an apricot silk kimono that Bill had thoughtfully packed before racing to the airport; brushed out my hair and tied it in an apricot ribbon. For the first time since my flight had begun its descent, I felt like myself.

When the nurse arrived with a wheelchair, I was a bit unnerved, but I had been in the hospital long enough to have had a bit of my ornery individuality subdued, and got aboard for the ride to the X-ray department. I joined the mass of patients on stretchers, in wheelchairs and in rows on long wooden benches. I felt a bit put out, since I thought my appointment meant that I had a special time reserved. My turn finally arrived, and an energetic technician zipped in and out of a shielded booth, positioning me for the exposure, running back in, calling "Hold your breath" and clicking a shot; then a measured "b r e a t h e" and then racing out of his safety booth again, to choreograph the next pose.

When I returned to my room it was filled with flowers—including some Bill had brought from our own garden. They dispelled the gloom that had crept back while I was waiting for X-rays, and I tumbled to the idea that the telephone by my bedside worked just like any other. There were still two hours until Bill, Dick and Stephanie would show up for lunch. I'd use the time to call my stepchildren, family and friends, to assure them personally that the ordeal was now over. Now and again a shadow of apprehension would blot my happiness, but a line out to a friend in the world where innards didn't have to be thought about, much less photographed, would soon get things bright again.

On the stroke of twelve, Bill, Dick and Stephanie bounded through the door laden with bags and baskets. They began to unpack a miniature restaurant. First a tablecloth was ceremoniously spread over a table they commandeered from a corridor.

Next, Jeff's china and flatware, cleaner than it had been in ages, I was quite sure. Then Bill produced a sorrel soup with a flourish, and Stephanie pulled out one of her marvelous quiches. Dick displayed an icy Chablis and we set to devouring the feast.

In all of the memorable meals we've shared, there was never one in which our love for each other was more a part of every morsel. In the short time between their leaving the hospital the day before, and closing time of the Georgetown shops, Bill and Stephanie had found everything they needed to equip a bachelor kitchen to cook a feast. Dick had scouted up one of my very favorite wines, and fresh strawberries for dessert. Bill cooked the soup at night, so it would be properly chilled for lunch, and Stephanie timed the quiche so that it was still piping hot when they got to my room. I had never eaten a meal with greater relish or joy than this one, which they had produced by putting aside their fears to allay mine. It was an interlude filled with magic.

We were finishing the strawberries when the doctor came in with the X-rays in his hand. One glance at his ashen face told us that the magic was all over.

# CHAPTER III

# Terror and Despair

The shadow on the X-ray hadn't been caused by an unreliable machine or a flaw in the film. It had been caused by a tumor in the lower lobe of my left lung, now perfectly visible in the unquestionably accurate plates produced by the hospital's main X-ray unit. "Our expert is quite sure that it is malignant." The doctor's voice penetrated into my stunned stupor from far away. "Surgery cannot be delayed."

I didn't hear much of the technical explanation of the way in which the tumor had cut the supply of oxygen to my heart and produced the heart attack symptoms. My mind fell off reality and into a whirlwind of terror. The only words that penetrated through the shrieking of the furies that swirled around me were "Malignant. Surgery. Survival." I grasped on those as comprehensible links to the world from which I had fallen, and tried to use them to pull myself back, but they only accelerated the spinning of the vortex.

Malignancy? In a body as strong and vital as mine? In a life in tune with nature? Impossible. Surgery? Violating the wholeness and balance with a knife? Possibly cutting away the very core of unity that gave me strength? Unthinkable. Survival? A real question about the possibility of being alive for much longer? Incredible. My life was sunshine and roses. All of these things could not be. But they apparently were. They were not mistakes, they were facts. And the understanding of those facts spun me along in a mindless panic. I needed to escape from the nightmare, but it had no walls to break through. The horrors had no forms or shapes to grip and fight. Instead they spread within and without, an amorphous, lethal, horrible vague cloud. My body and mind roiled, and past and present disappeared in a malevolent, convulsed kaleidoscope of hallucination that had become my future.

The whirlwind accelerated, and the roar of the wind became the scream of ten thousand voices that surely must be the sound of hell. My nightmare resolved to a vision of the tentacles of colonies of traitor cells spreading to engulf my body, reaching up to my head, growing to bloody nodules, the head screaming, joining in the solid sound of agony, then becoming the entire sound as the final horrible growths became the agony. And then silence. Like death after torment, a terrible quiet followed the primordial terror.

This was a different sort of unreality. I could see and hear and understand. But I refused to accept. It simply could not be true. Malignancy was a cosmic punishment reserved for those who had insulted their bodies with abuse or neglect. It couldn't be possible in a faithful child of nature. I had lived my entire life in reverence to nature's laws. Surely that meant that a calamity of this sort was impossible. It had to be a terrible mistake. The doctor was wrong. The X-rays had been mistaken a second time. Some other explanation had to exist.

Finally I came back to reality, and I saw the pallor of Bill's and Dick's faces. Their stunned horror broke through my madness and made me understand that I had cancer. Lung cancer. A very fast and almost invariably fatal disease. It was really so. I was really going to die soon. Perhaps by pieces. I wondered what it would be like to be sick. How I would feel as I disinte-grated. If death would finally come as a relief. And what it would be like to die—and to be dead.

I wondered, too, what it was going to be like for Bill and Dick, separated from me now by the tremendous chasm of life and death, for they were alive, pertained to life and living, and I was now under a sentence of death, with only the day and hour remaining to be filled in on the certificate. I was beyond any help they could offer. That chasm that separated me from Bill and Dick seemed to have cut me off from everything that had been central to my life. My harmony with nature, the charmed existence I had enjoyed, the vital appreciation of every minute, all were left over on the other side, and there was no way to return to them or to bring them over to the side I shared with my doom.

I began to feel something akin to embarrassment as I realized that I was bankrupt in an area in which I had previously enjoyed unlimited wealth. I had assumed perfect health as my natural condition. Strength to do and to enjoy had always been a basic fact of my life, but now the facts were changing. I could no longer count on the vigor to dominate problems, and I was faced with the gravest problem of all. I didn't know what resources would be left. Surely a strong spirit must exist in concert with a healthy body. The ability to laugh and work, my optimism, the capacity to find deep satisfaction in my relationships with the people I love—all must, to some extent, presuppose physical well-being. Everything in my life up to that point had presup-posed physical well-being. There might be nothing left with which to fight. Now, destitute of basic resources, I might be defenseless.

I remembered an article I once read about a lung cancer victim. The tortures he suffered as the disease dragged him to his death were so graphically portrayed that I became nauseated. I remember, too, the reproach and indignation I had felt because a human being had been afflicted with such an obscene indignity, and wondered now how much insult I would be called upon to bear. I recalled with shocking clarity a film to which I had taken Bill, a four-packs-a-day smoker, in the hope of getting him to stop poisoning his lungs. The effects of lung cancer were shown, step by inevitable step, from detection through disintegration to the death that occurs usually within six months—in 96 percent of all cases.

"It is by no means an absolute diagnosis," the doctor ventured. He had been frank about the probability that it was an accurate diagnosis, but wanted to leave us a bit of hope to help us through the next few days. The head of the department of pulmonary diseases of Georgetown University Hospital had a remarkable ability to diagnose tumors such as mine from X-rays. He had been called in by the cardiologist and had pronounced the terrible judgment. But there was an outside chance, very slim, but possible, that the tumor was benign.

I opted to cling to that chance. Not too tenaciously, and without too many illusions. But there just wasn't anything to do but hope or despair, and hope, the lifelong habit, offered a respite, a chance to marshal strength, time to buttress my emotions to meet onslaughts to come. Hope could build a bridge back to Bill and Dick, whom I'd left in the world of life. It would help hold all of our shattered nerves together and help us prepare ourselves to face the definitive answer which would come from a bronchoscopy, which would be performed in three days. I knew that the eminent professor who had diagnosed cancer in my lung was probably right. Almost definitely right. But although I knew that this was so I permitted myself to feel that it might not be, and reminded myself that 4 percent of lung cancer patients did survive.

The cardiologist explained the procedures for the next three days. Mostly electrocardiograms and other tests to determine whether or not my heart had stabilized enough for surgery. And the bronchoscopy, which sounded like a medieval torture. No anesthesia could be given, yet I had to maintain perfect stillness as a long flexible tube was pushed into my nose, through my esophagus and left bronchial tube, and into a pulmonary sack at the bottom of my left lung. Once there, a fluoroscopic scanner would help the doctor decide when to activate the small snippers at the end of the tube and cut off a piece of the tumor to pull back out for analysis. If the biopsy confirmed malignancy, and he was very sure that it would, we would schedule surgery as soon as possible, for time would be critically important. The doctor walked toward the door gently, almost whispering that he would see us tomorrow.

Suddenly, as if on cue, Bill and I burst into uncontrolled sobbing. He tightened his grip around me and we moaned, "No! No! No! No! No!" As our tears flowed down our faces, Dick screamed his own scream, silently, in his way. He embraced me and murmured: "You and Bill should have some time alone." Then he took my chin in his hand, as if he were the parent and I the child. "Please don't fall into despair," he urged gently. I nodded numbly as he left.

When we had finally cried out the torrent inside us, Bill and I fell into a deep stillness. Squeezing my hand, Bill said: "Dick is right. We mustn't fall into despair."

"I know," I answered. "Tears will only defeat us. Let's pledge to each other that these will be the last tears, no matter what happens."

"That's a lot to promise," Bill began to protest. "But no more tears." As he said it his eyes filled, but somehow the tears didn't fall. "I know you're going to make it," he told me softly. "And I think you know that, too." Then he kissed me and tucked the blanket up under my chin. "Now, you'd better take a nap."

The next day the panic was gone, and I began to feel my way around the very narrow limits of the world which was now mine. The open horizons, complete freedom and apparently unlimited strength of just a few days ago had become a future that might last no more than a few months, with very little peace of mind to use those months. Possibilities slammed shut, one after another. Harvests of gratifications, long and carefully tended toward a time when they would be enjoyed, withered.

My body and my health had been perfectly maintained all of my life, both for the pleasure of having them perfect and for the vigorous, active and joyful old age I had planned to have. My relatives had all lived into their late seventies and eighties, and I had planned to live even longer, and kept up my body with that old age in mind. I would never live it, and with that loss I felt the doors of decades of potential pleasures and experiences slam shut.

I would never play with a grandchild. I wouldn't see my son and Bill's children grow older and would be deprived of the satisfaction and pride of their growing accomplishments and contentments. I wouldn't be able to complete the natural course of my marriage with Bill. We had just assumed that it had much longer to run, that there was much, much more that had to be discovered and done. All these losses closed more doors, and closed my world in even tighter.

My career had been carefully pursued for many years, and was returning an ever-accelerating sequence of achievements, rewards and opportunities. Those would just disappear, for I did not work with tangible objects, but with concepts, which could not be inherited. My projects would die with me or before me. Those that had not been started would never begin. And more doors slammed.

When all of the doors had closed I was left in a small hall, perhaps six months long, with just that one terrifying door at the end. Just a little time, and virtually inevitable, very imminent, death. So much would never be experienced. So many joys never repeated. So little left. I wouldn't even have the blessing my parents had had of dying quickly after brief illnesses. My death would take some time, and I would probably be in a great deal of pain and incapacitated by the time I got to the end of the hall. I would also probably be a great burden for the people who would try to ease the trip. Bill would have to watch me disintegrate and suffer. He and Dick would probably come to hope for my death as they now hoped for my life, when I got so far along that my life would be a painful burden to me.

Yet they could not share in the terror I felt at the nearness of death. The awesome finality, the possibility of void and nothingness, the infinite emptiness that were part of my very infrequent contemplation of death took on a concrete immediacy which I believe can be had only from a close vantage point. I looked at the monstrous thing and shuddered. I was close enough to feel the chill as I peered into the deep velvety black and saw absolutely nothing.

Whether or not I was peering into my abyss, I was still a patient of the Georgetown University Hospital and, as such, would have to follow the routine which had been established when the first hospital cornerstone had been laid at the founding of the first hospital centuries ago: that the patient is the passive object of all activity, the doctors, nurses and staff the active subjects. I decided that it would be wasteful to use energy that would be desperately needed to fight my disease in simply asserting my personality, so I allowed myself to be trundled about, poked, prodded, kept waiting and rushed. The significant work went on around the mass of trivia. EKGs were taken and studied, and I got my briefing on the bronchoscopy procedure.

The bronchoscopy procedure is a minor operation performed with a long tube with a tiny snipping and gripping mechanism at the end. The tube is guided with the aid of a large fluoroscope, which projects on an overhead screen. Because the movement and direction of the tube must be assisted by small movements by the patient, no anesthetic is possible except for a local lacquer anesthetic sprayed on the throat just prior to inserting the tube.

The procedure would be performed while I sat in a dentist's-type adjustable chair, which coupled with the mobile fluoroscopy unit would permit locating and reaching the precise spot at which the surgeon must snip. I was told that I must not move in any way, except as instructed by the surgeon to help him get the snippers to their target. Finally, I was warned that the procedure would be taxing and extremely unpleasant.

One point had been made very forcefully in the briefing sessions: on the morning of the bronchoscopy I was not to consume anything. Not even a drop of water. "Don't even brush your teeth," they warned. "You might swallow some of the rinse water." I was naturally alarmed when, barely two hours before the porcedure was scheduled to begin, a nurse rushed in with a pint of some liquid for me to drink so that she could complete a sugar test prior to my release the following day. She had failed to complete the test the day before, as scheduled, and was interested only in covering her tracks. This was my first indication that I had to be prepared to protect my well-being from some of the people who were trying to cure me as well as from the disease itself.

The second indication that all peril did not lie with my cancer came right after the first. The surgeon and some nurses were in a flap when I was wheeled down a long hall to what I assumed must be the operating room. I was correct in my assumption, but it turned out that that was not my destination. In spite of the very ceremonious briefings, my dedicated rehearsals, and the surgeon's request that I permit student observers to be present, the operating room had not been reserved, and was being used when we tried to go in.

The occupied room contained the movable dentist's chair, the mobile fluoroscopy unit and, I presume, sufficient space for the gallery of students who were on hand to watch the operation. The fluoroscopy examining room in which the doctor decided to try to operate did not. It had a slab table and a stationary fluoroscopy unit. Two nervous members of the team gave me a briefing on the changes. Since the table and fluoroscopy unit couldn't move, I would have to.

Just as I had about absorbed the shock of the price of discomfort I would have to pay for someone's lack of attention to detail, the surgeon asked for the lacquer anesthetic. "Oops! I forgot it," chirped the nurse, who had been chatting with one of the young intern observers. "I'll be right back with it," and with that she popped out in pursuit of the forgotten drug. The surgeon was beginning to show some loss of composure, and I was horrified.

The doctor's composure slipped even further as the operation progressed. He barked commands, some of which seemed contradictory, to everyone. I hoped that his assistant and the fluoroscope operator knew what he wanted. I never figured out where "Here!" was, and finally one of the assistants was dragging me back and forth across the slab to duplicate the movements I assumed were readily available in the chair and fluoroscope intended for bronchoscopies.

The students whom the surgeon had asked me to permit in the operation didn't seem to notice the flap going on on our side of the room. The long Fourth of July weekend was coming up, and they were busily comparing flight plans for the holiday. A burst of excited chatter came when two of the "observers" discovered that they would be sharing the same flight, and laughter and the banter of schoolboys filled the room. It seemed the final indignity of a very unpleasant morning that these young doctors, whose presence their professor thought would be so rewarding, did not deign to pay attention to the proceedings but added their own touch to the debacle. I slowly raised my arm out toward them and brandished a fist. "Quiet!"

shouted the surgeon, but I kept the fist stretched toward them until they had all seen my fury at their callous contempt and stopped their chattering.

The operation went on far longer than I had been told it would, but the original schedule had been reckoned on the basis of the right equipment. Finally the now quite thoroughly ruffled surgeon made the snippet and ordered me to roll over on my side. A billow of bright red blood formed at my lips and it was over.

We had a month's grace period before my operation and had decided to spend it in the country, where we have always been happiest. We had completed a make-over of the house in the last year and a half, and I wanted to enjoy the fruits of our planning and labors. After years of dreaming, we had persuaded a sprite-ly octogenarian in a neighboring town to part with a two-century-old house that was collapsing on her property. Disassembled, the house became beams for our walls and ceilings, and exquisitely weathered paneling became a gigantic kitchen and a beautiful small study. Another eighty-year-old woman of prodigal energy and a genius for quilting made the patchwork that covered every piece of upholstered furniture, pieced together every pair of draperies, bedspreads, throw pillows and miscellany that brought our interior into more perfect rhyme with the turn-of-the-century decks and walkways, patios, gazebos and gardens outside.

As we swung into the driveway I got a tremendous jolt of joy at being back in the little world I had left ten days and an eternity ago. It seemed for one brief moment as if the horrible mistake had been discovered, the diagnosis corrected, the damage repaired, and that I could come back to life as I had always lived it here in the country with Bill.

I curled up on a chaise beside the French doors looking out onto the terrace where we had built a shelter for the cats who dropped by to be fed and watched them frolic. As I watched, the joy drained out of me, for there, amid all of the things dearest to me, I realized what I was about to lose and my complete helplessness at preventing that loss. The paradise that this house represented for Bill and me was slipping away, and I couldn't do a thing to stop it.

The next day more of my life slipped away as I began to call business associates to terminate projects or to relinquish my part of them. I disassembled my work over the course of that day, closing off dreams I had worked years to bring to reality.

The surgeon had not called with the results of the bronchos-copy several days after he had promised to be in touch with us. Bill and I called the hospital repeatedly, but none of the people who had been involved in that strange operation ever seemed available to come to the telephone or inclined to return our calls. Finally we spent an entire morning trying, and got through to one of the residents who had assisted. He promised to get the results to us, and at the end of the day the surgeon called to tell us that the results were inconclusive. It didn't seem possible that a biopsy could be inconclusive, but there it was. Perhaps the unusual conditions had made getting an accurate snip impos-sible, and I had endured the operation only to have a piece of an unaffected lobe analyzed.

The complete loss of control over my destiny drove me into a deep depression. But there was something else wrong, some other element out of place which I had not been able to identify. Something about the upcoming surgery made me especially anxious, in a way that did not relate to the direct life-or-death question which the surgery was intended to resolve. I could sense that, lost in the pile of events controlled by doctors, nurses and hospitals, there was something which I should be control-ling, and which I was not.

# CHAPTER IV

# Surgery, Futility and Doom

My plans for surgery had been made in haste and panic, and loose ends seemed to have been left in suspension at every step of the process. "Hurry, save yourself," my doctors urged. "Time is the name of the game." The Georgetown Hospital's cardiologists recommended the best surgeon in the area, and, when they found that he was on vacation, telephoned him on holiday to arrange for my operation on the morning he returned, August 5. Cardiac stress tests were scheduled for the day before, to be certain that my heart would be able to withstand the trauma of surgery. I was to go back to Georgetown on August 3.

The crucial decisions of my life seemed to be whirling around me, made by others, made on the basis of apparent expediency, made with no time for consideration, reflection, contemplation. And, most especially, made without much more than token participation by me. I was to entrust my life to a man I would not meet until the morning he was to operate on me. I might have to have the surgery while wired up to a heart monitor. Or the surgery might be ruled out by the cardiac stress test the day before. My heart might be too weak to permit the surgeon to eliminate the cancer and save my life. And I wouldn't know until the day before. I had never before made important decisions until I was completely ready and knew instinctively what was best for me. Now, I was being propelled into what might prove to be one of the most important—or even last—decisions of my life in a frenzy of anguish and doubt. Whether or not part or all of the procedure was best or even right wasn't even discussed. It was necessary and urgent to act quickly, without questioning the decisions which were being made for me.

A telephone call from Bill's sister, Jean, brought the frantic rush to a stop. "Do you think you'll be able to shuttle between Georgetown and New York for all of the postoperative care you're going to need?" she asked. Postoperative! My imagination and planning had stopped with the surgeon's knife. In the shock and urgency of discovering that I apparently had cancer we had not even considered that the ordeal didn't end with surgery, but really just began there, and that it would be impossible to commute for the treatments to follow from our home in New York.

Dr. Alfred Jaretzki III, at the top of his profession, had an office in the Columbia Presbyterian Medical Center. And he could see me at once, Jean reported.

The next afternoon Bill and I were shown into the sedative, impersonal blandness of the big waiting room, an ocean of beige where people sat becalmed. I leafed through a stack of hospital newsletters hoping to find some item on Doctor Jaretzki that I could mention to make our contact less impersonal, but there was nothing. I wanted communication and empathy with my surgeon. I needed a superman with impeccable credentials, of course. But also a wise, kind father whose concern would be an anodyne for my fears. I would ask Dr. Jaretzki to illumine the shadows for me, explain my malignancy. Why had it come so swiftly and in defiance of statistics? If he could find a clue in my past, he could guide me, be an ally in my recovery.

Wishing, hoping, I hardly noticed the receptionist when she came to take us to Dr. Jaretzki's office.

The kindly father fantasy evaporated. It was, indeed, a superman who rose to greet us. Dr. Alfred Jaretzki III radiated energy, power, authority, assurance . . . an almost visibly crackling aura of professional status and unapologetic consciousness of worth. He waited, at ease, for us to begin the conversation. We were suppliants at Parnassus.

After polite greetings Bill tried first contact. He'd noticed and appreciated the elegantly potted display in the office: velvety, perfect African violets, cyclamen, achimenes, all without a wilted leaf. Bill complimented the doctor on the plants. "My secretary has the green thumb," said Doctor Jaretzki in a tone that disclaimed both responsibility and interest. He reached for my bulging dossier of Georgetown records and X-rays. Bill and I looked at each other. The doctor very obviously did not want, and would not tolerate, a personal involvement of any sort with a prospective patient.

As he asked the usual health questions and scribbled my answers, I sat coolly erect, trying to match his crispness. But my voice rebelled. When he asked, "Do you smoke?" I heard my answer wobble, tremulous with protest, "I do not and have never smoked a cigarette in my entire life!" Behind it was the weight of the question I wanted so desperately to ask: I've followed all the rules of health and more, so how could this have happened to me?

Doctor Jaretzki looked at me dispassionately. My cancer wasn't his fault and sympathy is only a frill. "A good surgeon operates with his hands but never his heart." The quote from Dumas seemed to be embodied by the man facing me across the desk.

Quite a few questions later, the litany of negative answers I had given—no wheeze, cough, sputum, pain, tiredness, sensation of weight in the chest, nothing to alert me, nothing until that day on the plane—made me realize what extraordinary good health I had taken for granted.

"You do appear to be in excellent overall health."

"Then perhaps the tumor isn't malignant," Bill ventured, hoping aloud.

Doctor Jaretzki considered us. "Unfortunately, I believe that it is. Malignancy is almost a certainty with the density and conformation I see on the X-rays."

"And I'm in good health with a malignant tumor in my lung?"

He nodded. "It's odd, but in case after case it seems as if the individual is healthier and hardier than most, and yet cancer strikes like a thunderbolt."

I persisted. "Malignancy just doesn't square with the fact that I haven't had a headache in five years."

"You've had your recent symptoms," he answered. There would be no more speculation; we were dealing with an accomplished fact.

Our original date for surgery had been August 5; Dr. Jaretzki, checking his schedule, substituted Tuesday, August 6. I asked about the cardiac stress test.

"I am not a cardiologist, but I don't foresee a problem with it."

He was right, of course. The cardiac element had dwindled in importance with the shift from Washington to New York, cardiologists to surgeon. I finally took the test pedaling on a stationary bicycle in the cardiologist's office and got a full, unqualified clearance for surgery.

I asked Dr. Jaretzki to explain what we could expect from the operation.

"There are several possibilities. You must be prepared for any one of them."

He laid them out, neatly. The best we could hope for was that the tumor could be totally and cleanly excised. Or a portion of my lung might have to be cut away with the tumor. Or the entire left lung might have to be removed. Or the cancer might have metastasized and would then be inoperable and hopeless.

Bill and I considered the progressively grimmer choices as the doctor explained the process of biopsy: removing tissue from the tumor site during the operation and rushing it to the pathology lab to establish its malignancy. Initial biopsy confirms the surgeon's findings but does not indicate the strain of cancer involved. That is determined after several days of further lab work-ups, and the specific identification that emerges can indicate the kind of postoperative treatment a patient receives—and the patient's future prospects, since some cancers are more amenable to treatment and have higher rates of cure than others.

Dr. Jaretzki's terse presentation had a strange effect on me. I drew strength from it, even from his detachment as he offered me the obscene possibilities—cut clean, cut more, cut all, or too late for cutting. I had looked for communication with my surgeon and had been very firmly rebuffed. Now I felt a rapport with him. The rapport lay in what he *didn't* say, the sympathy he didn't offer, the complete lack of condescension. It was curious how much I'd trust a knife in his Olympian hands. I had faith in my surgeon's ego.

I wanted to engage private nurses. Bill emphasized that they must be "around the clock" for the duration of my stay.

"We'll arrange for it," Dr. Jaretzki said, seeming to dismiss the subject. He scribbled a note on his pad.

"But I must interview the nurses in advance—before they are hired," I persisted. "When and how can that be arranged?"

"That's entirely out of the question," the doctor waved the request aside. "We have no way whatever of knowing which nurses will be available until the appointed shift arrives," he explained, adding reassuringly: "However, on each shift the same nurse will then remain until your release, assuring continuity of care." Before I could burst out in protest he continued: "It's all handled by nurses' registry—they send whoever is available." I was dumbstruck.

"Do you mean that I shall have no control over the selection—and that I must take *pot luck*—that my care will be in the hands of individuals I have not even met before?"

"Our nurses are first-rate," the surgeon declared, clearly intending that this would end the discussion.

"What if she is indifferent? Or a slob? Or a fiend? I will have to make some private arrangements," I began to plan aloud. "I'll have the nurses brought in from the outside."

"I assure you," he said, without disguising his amusement, "that our nurses at Columbia are the best imaginable. And you cannot bring in others who would be unfamiliar with Columbia Presbyterian procedures. You would do yourself a great disservice even if it could be done. The nurses that you will have will be highly qualified and familiar with our systems. That's what you need most. Don't worry about their personalities."

"Well, in that case," I announced, "I shall bring my assistant—at least for the day shift for the first three or four days."

"What in the world *for?*" Dr. Jaretzki inquired incredulously.

"To coordinate things," I replied. "To see that everything flows smoothly and, frankly, to superintend the nurses. You see," I added by way of explanation, "it will be the first time in my life, that I can recall, that I shall be helpless and I've got to organize my own team."

Alfred Jaretzki III laughed a surprisingly loud and spontaneous laugh. I almost expected his receptionist to come running in at the sound. When he had resumed his professional gravity, he came around his desk, bent over me, and touched my shoulder. His manner, though still far from fatherly, seemed to show that my human absurdity had touched him in a way my human tragedy had not.

I had two weeks until surgery. Bill and I did what we have

always done, perhaps drawing a bit more out of each shared joy but living our familiar life. And it was not just a time of waiting, it was a time of preparation. In nature's order, I was finding my own. From nature's solace I was taking strength. It had always been so when I needed to reach inside myself to find resources, marshal courage and understanding, but never so much as now. Some primordial memory sent me to the sea, the Atlantic beaches near our home. I wanted cleansing, I wanted the wash of tides to clear the whirling confusion in my mind so that I might begin to examine my situation. Two weeks to go. Two weeks to decide what August 6 could mean to my existence; what would be asked, no, *demanded* of me. The pounding Atlantic waves gave me power to clear my mind and I sat alone for hours on a high dune gazing into white rolling water. I felt as I had in childhood, when a wet, icy compress cooling my fevered forehead made me simultaneously shudder with chill and murmur with delight. Slowly clarity came. Clarity lost since that disastrous day in June. Clarity which showed what must be done. Not the decision on surgery that was long since out of my hands. But my contribution to it.

There is someting I have always done which I call "mental rehearsal." Over the years, I've perfected a technique of learning to do a thing by living it mentally, every detail in advance, before it becomes actuality. I experience it over and over before it happens. As a child, I spent summers with my family at a lake, and each Sunday, as we'd row across it, my father would slip out of the boat for a mid-lake swim. I remember wanting to copy the smooth, strong strokes he used in the water. Even though I hadn't yet learned to swim, I thought I could learn, could absorb his skill into myself by intensely concentrating on how he did it. My leg muscles flexed in his rhythm, my shoulders moved to his motions, and though I'd been sitting in the boat while he swam, I was exhausted when we reached shore! I concentrated on the repetition of the performance each night in bed for a week. I saw myself swimming, I felt myself swimming until even the rhythmic twitches of my muscles became unnecessary and I could lie perfectly still, experiencing each sensation fully in my mind. I was so sure of what I felt that on the next Sunday, when my father began his swim, I asked to join him. He readied himself to be my water-wings, his hands under my stomach, but I slid from his grasp and struck out, swimming. There was no fear or strangeness. I swam because I knew I was ready, knew I could do it.

Since that day in the summer lake, I've used my "mental rehearsal" for many things: learning to figure skate, to drive a stick-shift car and years later in business. I knew I needed it now. I would have to ask Dr. Jaretzki to tell me every expected procedure from the moment I entered the hospital on the evening of Sunday, August 4, through the operation on Tuesday and afterwards, when I emerged from anesthesia. I would memorize hospital routines, practice the exercises now, thoroughly learn the drill, anything to assist in my own recovery, to make it happen faster. I had to know now, for the pre-knowledge would be my only armor against whatever the surgery revealed. I must be prepared.

I called Dr. Jaretzki for an extra consultation. He kept asking, "Why do you have to know that now? What possible good can it do you?" But when I explained my need for detailed knowledge in terms of what would happen to me, he gave me the minutiae I needed.

"You don't like to be surprised, Mrs. McGrail."

"No, Doctor, I don't."

And so there was just one surprise on the night before surgery. After I had bathed and gotten ready to go to sleep a woman in hospital whites rushed in brandishing a razor. I remembered the pint of liquid the nurse had tried to get me to drink right before my bronchoscopy in Georgetown, and had visions of being mistakenly wheeled off for brain surgery or a hysterectomy, as the woman obviously meant to shave me. "I am not to be shaved!" I protested. "I'm here for a thoracotomy." But it seemed that she was right, as unvarying hospital procedures indicated that I must have my chest and side shaved. She scraped away and actually did find some stray fuzz to justify the effort.

My shave provided a light note when Bill called to wish me a good night. When we'd hung up I settled back to absorb the roomful of flowers that he had brought in from the country. At nine a nurse came by to see if I hadn't changed my mind about taking a sleeping pill.

"No," I said, "I really don't want one." "But it is very important that you get a good night's sleep," she coaxed. "I'll sleep like a lamb," I reassured her. And I knew I would. For between the tests and visits and flowers I had drawn on an old store of tranquility that day. I transported myself to the beautiful mountain of vacations long past. Cherished sights, sounds, sensations, tastes and fragrances caressed me with loving re-membrance: dogwood blossoms and mountain laurel bloomed in the memory of my spirit, the icy ecstasy of wading the brook refreshed me even as then; while the thrill of the taste of sun-ripe berries seemed so real I thought that my fingertips were stained purple. The sweet honeysuckle fragrance that lingered in my imagination surpassed even the reality of jasmine that tumbled in its tub at my bedside. When it was time to sleep, I slept the sleep of my childhood in the mountain. At dawn I awoke refreshed and serene and slipped into the canvas surgical boots and crisp white muslin surgical gown that the nurse held out for me. I felt a deep poise. A serene confidence. It was a gift from the past. I was prepared for anything that was fated for this day. En route to surgery, I asked to see the sunrise. The attendant obliged, wheeling my stretcher to a luminous east window. It was a beautiful August morn. But the sky was like a strawberry froth. A childhood ditty ran through my mind and a faint shudder ran through me like a quiver of electricity: "Red skies in morning . . . sailors take warning."

I had determined days before that I would gain consciousness—even fleetingly—so that I could ask Dr. Jaretzki the verdict when he stopped by the recovery room immediately after the operation. He seemed to be a wavy mirage as I peered into the direction of his face. "Please tell me," I managed to stammer with a prodigious effort. And even in my dazed condition I realized that it had not gone well. He would have been exultant if he had excised it—even with part or *all* of the lung. But he said, "Never mind now—I will talk to you when you are out of the anesthesia and feeling stronger."

When my eyes and mind focused again, a spirited corps of young faces were urging me on to rally. I was being clapped briskly and commanded to cough . . . "harder" . . . "more" . . . "That's it, good!" "Breathe." "Blow up the balloon." Every command was more impossible than the one preceding it, but I knew that it was imperative to execute each drill. It was vital to recovery. Recovering from surgery would be more terrible now because the pain of the knife had been in vain! But no matter. I was determined to fight as staunchly to recover as if postoperative recovery were an end in itself. A strong, swift recovery. I will face whatever has to be faced after that. The first phase: recovery and only recovery. "Cough." "Breathe." "Blow the balloon." Excruciating. Impossible. But I will do it.

When I found myself in my room I was only half aware of where I was. A gentle face in starched white cap hovered over me and spoke in a sympathetic, competent voice. Thank heavens for this wonderful nurse, I thought. I held out my hand and she held it with compassion and sincerity. I felt I was going under again—but not before becoming aware of a terrible rigidity and pain in my upper torso. The next time I opened my eyes,

Bill was standing beside my bed—"Sweet baby," he was whispering—but he was soon out of focus and his voice faded away. And so it was for all of that first day. Troubled, dazed sleep; whenever I awoke the nurse brought me a bedpan and coaxed me to "try." But urinating seemed something that I would never be able to manage again. She might as well have asked a lamppost to urinate. Everything in me seemed rigid. But finally a few drops trickled into the pan. I signaled for her not to take it away—I wanted to try for a more respectable yield. But after what seemed to be an eternity of straining, she gently removed the bedpan and said we'd try later. It was a very good sign. I remembered Dr. Jaretzki's advice when he briefed me on the optimum-response-performance profile of postoperative patients. Natural urination was high on the list. Not only was the pain and discomfort of a catheter eliminated that way—but the spontaneous resumption of the function augured well for healthy resumption of other vital bodily functions. It seems odd that my total and transcending concentration could be focused on urinating, yet I was completely absorbed in the task.

The next morning Dr. Jaretzki arrived promptly at eight as he had promised. His face was pale, the suntan he wore yesterday seemed to have drained away. There was a trace of melancholy in his demeanor but no indication of emotion. I smiled and said "Good morning" and he smiled a greeting as he sat down beside my bed. "I am sorry to have to tell you . . ." The tumor was indeed malignant and it had metastasized. Two nodules touched on the pericardium (the lining of the heart). It was, as I had sensed in that fuzzy moment in the recovery room, inoperable. The tumor was still inside my lung. Large as a golf ball. I had been carved open, mutilated, and lay here now in indescribable pain—*in vain*. "I considered it too early to tell you and I wanted to wait a few days," he confessed, "but your husband and your son gave me an ultimatum: either I told you at once— or they would."

Yes, I nodded. "They promised me that nothing at all would be kept from me—that I would know everything as soon as they knew. They understood that I would have to know at once." I looked at the surgeon squarely. " *You* had promised me, too. Wouldn't you have kept your promise?"

"I would have kept it, but not so soon."

"And what would you have told me in the meantime?"

It didn't seem in keeping with his straightforward, matter-of-fact character, but apparently Dr. Jaretzki had planned to feed me pablum, for a guilty expression replaced the usual self-assurance as he answered a shade defensively: "It isn't as if knowing as of this very minute could help you in any way."

"You're wrong, Doctor. It could help me in every way. How could I begin to cope if I weren't aware of all of the facts?"

"Cope?" Dr. Jaretzki relaxed and even half smiled. "You have enough to cope with at the moment," he said as he gestured in the direction of my bandaged torso, intravenous paraphenalia and drainage tubes.

Even though my glimmer of hope had vanished, even though the operation had been a catastrophic futility, I was surprised at the strength I felt surging through me. Reinforcement from every healthy cell, a synchronism of mind and body and whatever comprises the human spirit. It wasn't just emotional strength to bear the burden of the cancer, it was positive strength surging up to do battle for my life. I would fight! And I wanted my doctor as my ally.

"I understand what you have been telling me, Doctor, but I am going to fight for my life with every possible weapon . . ."

"Of course you are."

". . . including my own imagination."

"Well, imagination isn't much of a weapon against cancer. But we have the established courses of treatment, radiotherapy and chemotherapy. Once we have the pathology report on your carcinoma, we'll be better able to prescribe."

"But both of those therapies inflict terrible damage on healthy tissue, devastate the body almost as much as the disease," I protested.

"We are concerned with unhealthy tissue."

"There must be something else somewhere, or perhaps something I could do that would make a difference."

He was impatient now; I could see that he was not going to join me in exploring any new approaches.

"Mrs. McGrail, there is nothing in the world that you can do except undergo the prescribed course of cobalt and chemotherapy treatments. Without them, you wouldn't last long enough to try some of the other theories you seem so determined to find."

"Of course I'll do whatever is necessary, but . . . are there ever remissions of cancer without these standard treatments?"

"Absolutely."

"What!"

"Individuals have been known to have total remissions of cancer without any treatment whatever. Others have made an accommodation with the disease. They coexist with it, apparently without harm, perfectly able to coexist with the malignancy—without discomfort or apparent peril."

"My God," I shouted and felt for the first time during this discussion he sharp stabbing reminders of what lay beneath my mummy wrappings. "Then cancer can be cured!"

"I didn't say that!" the surgeon protested emphatically. "It's not a cure—there have been mysterious spontaneous remissions of cancer, or accommodations with it, so that both the individual and the cancer exist, as it were, each in its own place. No one can fathom how or why." I could see that he was sorry that he had gotten ensnared into this topic but I wanted desperately to keep him on this thrilling track.

I repeated almost inaudibly: "Then cancer can be cured."

"I must repeat," Dr. Jaretzki said sternly, "that I didn't say that."

"I know, but you did say that it can vanish spontaneously, leaving a patient free of cancer. That's a cure."

"What good is such talk?" the exasperated doctor said, sighing, "since we don't know how to accomplish it!"

"Ah, but it has been accomplished, and I never knew that before." Apparently there was something I could do that could make the difference! If one solitary human being had found a way back from malignancy without radioactive therapy or chemotherapy, then I could hope. Something had to be restored, reunited, rebuilt or redirected inside of me.

Dr. Jaretzki wouldn't humor me any longer. "You must be realistic. You cannot count on whimsy. You face a vicious killer!"

Our conversation was over. He had shocked me into an awareness of the bleakness of my chances, but I couldn't forget that spontaneous cures existed. I would take the regular cancer therapies, and I wanted to get to them right away, but if they didn't bring results I was going to look further, even into unproven research if that showed promise. Somewhere there was another way. I would try to find it.

Rapid postoperative recovery was my immediate goal. I was up on my feet the second day. I stretched my arms high over my head and slowly dropped them to my side in a tracing of a circle even before the physical therapist came to work with me, for I had been rehearsing mentally for a full day. On the second day I also managed to flip over to my right side from flat on my back. It had been impossible to simply roll over. Rigid, unyielding muscles refused. Then I remembered Dr. Jaretzki's boast: "You're going to feel as if the slightest stir will burst your incision wide open—but don't worry, when I sew you up you can play football and remain intact." He was right. Unable to negotiate the turn by simply turning over to my right, I flung myself up in the air like a whale leaping out of water and twisted my body in mid-fling, landing on the right side. On the third morning I insisted on washing up by myself. The nurse begged me to allow her to sponge me in bed. ''Absolutely not.'' So she helped me into the bathroom. She set up a chair, small stool and night table containing my toiletries and handed me some un-reachable object if I needed it. It took almost three-quarters of an hour to sponge bathe out of a basin, dry, brush my teeth, wash my face, and apply makeup, comb my hair, spritz on a cloud of cologne and slip into a fresh gown. It was exhausting and I napped for a half-hour after completing this daily ritual. Some mornings in the first few days after surgery I would be covered with sweat when I finished my ritual. Then, the nurse would do a touch-up sponging in bed. The regimen paid hand-some dividends. Although tired and spent after the ordeal, as soon as I rested I felt aglow with life and achievement. And not the least of it was that I looked and felt attractive and well-groomed all day. It gave me a lift, and Bill, Dick and his wife were thrilled with the fact that I ''looked so marvelous.'' They related my recovery progress to this visual and encouraging sign that I was as strong as an ox. I did not think of long-term recovery. Only of the best possible postoperative recovery. I made rules and did not deviate from them. There would be no visitors except my immediate family, no changes in my daily routine. My energies were all directed toward recovery and that took every moment of my waking time.

My family's visits brought love and laughter into my room and their banter made it impossible for me to feel threatened, let alone doomed. My nurses, as Dr. Jaretzki had predicted, gave me kind, expert care. The hospital personnel, the therapists from the Pulmonary Department of Columbia University all urged me on like good fight managers, putting me through all the physical paces necessary to recovery. So much caring, so much help! But it was all for recovery from the surgeon's scalpel. After that the cancer treatments would begin.

"You need to cry. Let yourself go and be human." I think Doctor Jaretzki felt I was hurting myself by holding back tears. But I would not. I asked if mine was one of the "luckier" cancers, and was there hope that radiotherapy and chemotherapy could shrink the tumor?

"That's impossible to predict."

"But if it did, could I calculate in months or years?"

He answered noncommittally, "If you are alive six months from now, I'll be better able to assess the situation."

Then I asked, "Is there anything I can do right now besides the treatments?"

He looked at me without flinching. "You can make your will. And you can go home and do the things you have wanted to do all of your life."

# CHAPTER V

# Acceptance and Determination

I was home again, back in the dappled sunshine of the gazebo, where I'd found tranquil moments of happiness even in the storm of confusion and anxiety between finding that I definitely did have cancer and surgery. The beauty of the place, in the center of our favorite plantings and elevated just a bit so that even the highest, healthiest plants didn't block the view of the others, always filled me with a quiet contentment.

The gazebo was filled with beautiful associations, too. Breakfasts with Bill, picnic lunches with weekend guests and friends, reunions with our children when they breezed in from their various corners of the world and, perhaps most fun of all, an occasional quiet lunch for just Bill and me.

We were having one of these quiet lunches together. Bill had brought out French bread, cheese, a crisp salad and white wine. The table was heaped high with flowers, and the garden was bursting with beautiful blooms. But for all of the beauty and all of the pleasures that were there for me, I found no joy or comfort in the gazebo that day.

I was preoccupied with my cancer, still within me, still consuming my body and my life. It seemed that I could actually feel the lump deep within my rib cage as I compulsively stroked the area of the incision. I felt disassociated, alien, with a touch of double vision making my most familiar and dearest surroundings look strange.

I had looked forward to coming to the gazebo after the futile surgery to find whatever I needed to face the new reality of my life, but everything was wrong. The lunch Bill prepared had no savor. The sunlight brought no warmth. The place itself was not permeated with contentment as it had always been before. Everything was wrong. No. I was wrong! I realized that I had lost myself to despondency and that that was why nothing seemed right. I had become so preoccupied with the apparent inevitability of imminent death that nothing, not even our little paradise, could reach me through the gloom. For the first time in my life I was defeated and hopeless.

I realized that cancer had attacked my spirit as devastatingly as it had attacked my body, and that I had to fight and defeat that assault on my spirit before I could begin to defend my body, for my spirit would be the strongest weapon in my body's defense. I would draw my strength from the things I loved. From Bill and our life together, from the house in the country and the things we had planted there, from the joys of times shared with friends and family. I must not let fear rob me of my best hope for prolonging my life—my real life, as a happy, fulfilled human being, not simply the state of being alive, or an absence of death.

And so I began to fight to bring my spirit back to vigorous health from the state to which fear had reduced it. I decided to make some conditions and rules for whatever life I had left, so that I would have the personal strength to do whatever was necessary to fight the disease of my body, and so that I would be able to really enjoy the time that was to be available to me—

whether that time was to be a few months or half a century.

I decided that the procedures that had brought me success in my personal and business life would be the ones to follow now. They had worked for me before, I knew them well and I had confidence in them. The first step was order. What were the goals? What resources were available to reach those goals? What path should I follow?

I already knew the goals: to regain my capacity to enjoy life and to do everything in my power to prolong my life. I had already met the obstacles: the disease of cancer that raged through my body and the fear of cancer that weakened my spirit. The resources were those I had always counted on: confidence, energy, imagination, perseverance, cheerfulness and—most difficult of all to use now—a closeness to nature.

Confidence was going to be needed first, and I was going to need a lot of it. I had to believe that my goals were attainable, and in my absolute right to be saved, my uniqueness and my value. I would need to believe that the bleak picture that Dr. Jaretzki had painted had a bright spot somewhere, and that bright spot was the key to survival. I would also need a very healthy ego to trust my own instincts, follow my own mind to a survival my doctor didn't seem to think was possible.

Primitive energy and vital force enable starfish to regenerate lost rays and crabs to grow new claws to replace missing parts. Human beings can't yet repair damaged parts through regeneration, but we can regenerate enthusiasm, optimism and drive in our own behalf. Energy is the catalyst that turns courage and will into action. I would use it to keep from being turned into "patient," the passive object of others' actions and concerns. I would be "person" doing all I could for myself.

Imagination would have two roles to fill for me. It would have to be used to try to develop alternative solutions to the problem which I had been assured on excellent authroity had no solution. I had to visualize success—see it clearly. And the more I saw it, the longer and closer I looked in my imagination, the better chance I had of pre-visualizing the direction in which a solution might lie. The second use would be as an anesthetic against the unavoidable pain I knew was coming. I would so completely project myself out of the very unpleasant situations I knew I must face into memories of happier times that the sensations of those happier times would prevail over the discomfort.

Perseverance has always worked to my good advantage. I had sometimes waited for years to bring some project to fruition, far beyond the point at which a reasonable person might have stopped trying. But that extra effort, the perseverance resulted in successes where reasonable people would have met failure. I would need to go beyond the point where reasonable people would have met failure. I would need to go beyond the point where reasonable people would stop. (In fact, making lists and plans to fight a disease after being given six months to live might already be in the unreasonable area.) I would have to deal with many defeats before I could expect to reach the success that might be beyond reason. I would have to ''Keep on keepin' on'' as the gospel song says, but that had been a habit for quite a while.

Cheerfulness was not something I could maintain by myself. It would have to be a reciprocal effort with the people near me. We couldn't let ourselves be trapped in a web of despair or we would never get out of it. We had to keep things light and upbeat, and I decided to make generating that mood my special responsibility.

My closeness to nature seemed to be a horrible joke at this point, a false relationship pretended by a cruel prankster to build my sense of security high for a spectacular fall. I had first refused to believe that I had been ''cursed'' or ''abandoned'' by nature. Then I believed that I had been, and that the process was irreversible. I found the patience and control to come back to a true understanding of nature, most especially its absolute lack of concern for the individual of any species from protozoa to people. The completely neutral majesty of nature, its laws without allowance for mitigating circumstances, its unswerving pursuit of its own epochal goals had been the center of my awed fascination. I had to recapture that awareness and try to use the might of the force I felt I could understand to help me rather than being intimidated into submission to cancer because I had felt that the force was actively against me.

I had taken my inventory and found that I had the same resources I had always counted on. Nothing had miraculously been added to my capacities, and I would try to see that nothing was lost to panic or despair. That set of qualities certainly doesn't represent a universal standard for the characteristics needed to fight cancer. They are just the ones I have. As anyone in the situation I faced must, I determined how to use my qualities to my best advantage.

The next step was to make plans for action I could take to help myself. I developed eleven rules to guide me:

1. I will follow doctors' orders, but never blindly, never rejecting the testimony of my own instincts, never doing what my instincts tell me to avoid.

2. I will take the standard treatments the doctors offer, take them gladly, but also look beyond them, since the final solution to cancer is still unknown. I will track down science and wisdom concerning cancer—whether it's evidence, a theory or embryonic but promising research—anywhere in the world. I will search out every possible clue, ask anyone and everyone until I reach my goal.

3. I will seek out nature's remedies as well and follow my own instincts in applying some of my natural healing persuasions. I will try to help myself each day, even in the smallest ways.

4. I will meet each development with grace and dignity.

5. I will not only remember to smile and laugh in reaction to others but I will make occasions for laughter myself.

6. I will not let discouragement sap my spirit and I will be on guard against the blues, no matter how momentary or innocent.

7. I will continue to generate hope for my family and friends, knowing that it is not enough that they hope for me, I must also give hope to them. Together we can defeat the void that would exist if my hope and cheer visibly waver.

8. I will not indulge in self-pity and I will not accept pity from any source, only good wishes.

9. I will not weep, even when I am alone I will not weep, for tears would deplete me and destroy the energy I need.

10. I will concentrate on living, not dying, never wasting one precious moment rehearsing for the grave. And I will hold the same stance in public and private, with others and when I am alone.

11. I cannot allow my cancer to become the dominating force in my family's life. Though a tremendous effort will certainly be required, we must try to live as normally as before, still seeking our joys where we have always found them: in each other, with friends, in hobbies, pipedreams and the endless kaleidoscope of wonders we have always seen in nature.

I had set my goals, marshaled my resources and planned my actions. Now it was time to begin. The first step was to get back to really enjoying my life. To make every day a marvelous day—whether it was to be my last or whether there would be thousands more.

Each day began with a breakfast ritual. I made certain that the croissants were perfectly warm. The soft-cooked eggs were done for exactly three minutes. Strawberry preserves were at room temperature, not refrigerator-cold. The table always had fresh flowers. Breakfast became a delicious pleasure of perfect details and perfect enjoyment. And it gave every day a positive start.

When we were in the city I used every opportunity to revisit the spots I really love. I stared soberly at the stolid yak in the Central Park Zoo, and giggled at the cavorting seals as they went through their deliberate, outrageous act. I trekked up to Yorkville to buy a mettwurst and to enjoy the acres of sausages hanging in the German butcher shops. I watched the chaste, correct waterfall in Paley Park, and observed people actually become more polite as they entered the little oasis of elegance and pleasant formality in the middle of the city.

I decided to brush up my Italian, and was chagrined at how much of the language I had lost through neglect. Bill and I had gone to evening courses for what seemed like ages just for the fun of speaking the musical language of a place whose melodies and rhythms we loved. Several years of neglect left me without enough to brush up. This loss was a lesson, for facilities other than language could certainly be lost through disuse. I resolved not to rob myself of any shred of identity because I neglected part of myself in preoccupation with survival. I resolved to live my life fully while I survived.

Each book, each play, each concert, art exhibit, dinner guest, meal and wine would now be chosen with infinitely greater care, a habit I soon wished I had developed decades earlier. Books, plays, and the like had always been limited commodities, priceless in their irreplaceability. A book read meant that another was not. Each choice eliminated other possibilities. I had never realized this so clearly, and had made many very lazy choices. My life would be improved by my insistence on choosing only the finest. I filled my time with joy and left no room for negative feelings.

I realized that filling my time with joy was a sacred obligation, since I was going to have to buy that time with pain. It would be a sacrilege to suffer to prolong my life and then squander on frivolities the time I had gained through suffering. I was prepared to enjoy life and to live it happily. My spirit was strong and I was ready now to renew the battle to save my body.

# CHAPTER VI

# The Brutalization of Cells and Psyche

The next step in the battle against the disease that was ravaging my body was a meeting with the radioactive therapist and the chemotherapist who had been called in by Dr. Jaretzki. I was to be briefed on the nature of the treatment I was about to receive and the possible side effects. I had dreaded this interview and the devastating treatment that would follow.

The radioactive therapist was a kind woman whose compassion surfaced during our discussion of the twenty-five sessions of deep radiation I would have. The treatment involved bombarding me with 5,000 rads—5,000!—and I'd read that one rad alone could inflict enough damage on body tissue to constitute a year of aging. Well, no help for it, but there was one thing I had to know.

"Doctor, I realize that the radioactive treatment will be directed at my lung, but since the tumor nodules touch on the lining of the heart, does that mean that my heart will be in the line of the beam?"

"Yes."

Yes? Then I might survive the cancer only to die of a weakened, prematurely aged heart. But I could not, must not pursue that line of thought, for if I did I would send these therapists with their rehearsed voices and careful eyes away, and I had sworn to do whatever had to be done without giving in to fear.

What side effects, I asked, could I expect from the radiation treatments?

The doctor's answers were general; I'm sure she gave them often. The intensity of side effects varied but I could expect ''nausea, loss of appetite, loss of energy, possible depression or malaise.'' In her neutral phrasing it sounded like the aftermath of a bad bout of flu. But still, her eyes kept shifting away from mine and today I realize that it was because of the questions I should have asked but didn't, the information I should have had about the long-term effects, the hidden subversion, the devastation of my body, treatment-induced, that would come to light considerably after the radioactive therapy. Perhaps she thought I might not live long enough to meet these complications—I don't know—but I didn't ask and she didn't volunteer.

''What is the optimum result I can hope for after completing the twenty-five sessions?''

''A total shrinking and scarring of the tumor.'' How often she must have answered that desperate question.

''And how will we know the result?''

''Periodic X-rays.''

My schedule, she explained, would be 5,000 rads over a period of 36 days for 25 actual treatments to the left lung, alternating between an erior and posterior lung at a depth of 9 centimeters. The flat calm of her approach helped me accept the knowledge that the only way to even a very precarious recovery would be a wholesale slaughter of healthy tissue along with the diseased.

In contrast, the glib chemotherapist spoke enthusiastically about his specialty. According to him, he had no bad news. Yes, he said, while it was true that chemotherapy was not entirely selective, it was still amazingly targeted toward destroying the malignant cells with side effects that were limited only to other fast-growing cells such as bone marrow, blood and hair.

His cheery tone was hard to bear. Only blood and bone marrow and hair cells plus whatever the X-rays would kill! Clearly, these combined treatments would be as surgical as my operation; parts of me would have to die so that other parts with higher life priorities might continue to exist. I had a flash of myself as a walking jigsaw puzzle of dead bits and pieces that still functioned.

"Don't worry," said the chemotherapist. "It will all be carefully controlled." And he added, with peculiar confidential intensity, almost for my ears alone, "We're going to take very good care of you."

And what would that be?

"In your case, Mrs. McGrail, the best combination to combine with the radioactive therapy would be Cytoxan and Ontavin."

Cytoxan sounded vaguely familiar to me. "What is Cytoxan?"

"Nitrogen mustard gas."

At once, unbidden, I remembered my father's stories about the poisonous killer of World War I and of the men who were gassed and survived lingering, many years later, in hospital wards. I, who wouldn't take medicines because they were chemicals, who didn't use aspirin because they were artificial, now forced to take mustard gas to save my life! "We must begin treatment at once," the chemotherapist said.

"At once?"

"We'll start in three days."

Three days! I was not ready to be changed beyond hope in three days!

"What is the procedure?" I managed to ask.

"It's done as an intravenous infusion. You will return for treatment every six weeks until you have had a total of seven infusions. Each infusion will take three and a half hours."

Three days later a young resident entered my hospital room pushing an intravenous rack. I knew him, I liked him. He had lank handlebar mustaches which made his expression dolorous and he was wearing wooden clogs. Had he always worn them? Perhaps I'd been too busy before with postoperative drills to be aware of the noise they made but now I was terribly alert, my eyes fixed on the intravenous rack, its pouch already filled with colorless liquid; swaying, suspended, waiting for me. But where was my chemotherapist? The young resident explained that the chemotherapist selected the combination of drugs to be given to a patient, but the infusion itself was left to a resident or nurse following orders. He himself was to give me my treatment right now. That was a surprise, but nothing like the second surprise that came out of our casual conversation. I found out about the ABC options open to the chemotherapist and the ABC procedure itself!

According to the resident, one out of every three cancer patients on chemotherapy gets the most potent combination of chemicals in the current arsenal. That patient is A. Patient B gets another combination of chemicals under study. But patient C (C-for-control) only thinks he is getting chemotherapy. Actually, in terms of chemical effectiveness, he is given a placebo. He is left on his own, at the mercy of the disease, to serve as a control to check against which the effectiveness of "A" and "B" are measured.

This came as a visceral shock, a numbing glimpse into a world of clinical science I cannot begin to understand. I know that there is no positive cure for cancer and thus all treatment is speculative. I can understand that there is no way of determining the most effective form of chemotherapeutical anti-cancer treatment unless ABC experimentation continues. But this knowledge is withheld from the cancer patient, because even if volunteers to omit the best treatment could be found, the simple fact that they were aware that they were not getting medicine could invalidate the research. There is a persistent theory about the emotional origins of cancer and the possible effectiveness of the body's own psychological defenses reinforced by the conviction that a cure is being given. Where would that factor be if a patient knew he was selected as a C? There are certainly unexplained remissions—some people do recover from cancer without medical intervention through mysterious inner resources of their own—but it seems a cruel hoax to offer bogus treatment in the interest of experimentation to people fighting for their lives.

Was that why the chemotherapist had assured me so confidentially that they'd "take good care of me"? My cancer was widespread, had metastasized. Surely I'd be getting the most potent poison-cure and I was grateful.

"This will hurt," said the young resident, as he put the intravenous needle into the large vein of my right wrist. The needle was taped in and then the wrist itself taped to a board. The clear liquid began to drip as soon as the tube was opened. And as I closed my eyes, settling in for the long wait, I heard the resident leave the room. I was glad he had not tried to "comfort the fearful patient." It wouldn't have worked.

Alone, I watched the droplets slide into the tube. Why had they left me alone? Suppose something went wrong? I wrestled with my demons not knowing that I wasn't in danger, not knowing that the liquid now in the pouch was only glucose and that the actual chemical infusion would come after my body had absorbed enough glucose to "take it." I realize that the cruelty of the omission was unintentional, but so many things that happen to patients in hospitals are cruelly unnecessary. I might have relaxed if I had known I still had time before the irreversible process began.

When the pouch was three-quarters empty, the young resident returned. He checked the suspended pouch, stopped the flow momentarily, then inserted a hypodermic needle into the pouch and emptied the vial attached to the needle. "You have only three-quarters of an hour to go,"he reassured me, with a good-luck pat on the shoulder. Then he called in a nurse to watch me and left again.

In fifteen minutes my stomach began to twist with unbelievable nausea and a rising tide of fluid filled my nose and mouth. I vomited, again, again, and again. Green bile spilled from my mouth—more—still more, as I continued to convulse and vomit. My eyes streamed helpless tears, the cold gluey sweat ran, congealed, burst forth again. I lost control of everything, every function as my insides rebelled completely, and my nerves danced with stabbing fire. "Can't you . . . give . . . me something . . . make it stop?" I begged the nurse. As I writhed and vomited, she ran for the resident. He appeared at once and spoke to me. I tried to pay attention as best I could from somewhere inside my retching, quivering misery. I had already been given something against nausea, he said. I'd been given Compozine, more familiar as a tranquilizer but expected to control a violent reaction like this. Only it hadn't! "Sometimes," said the resident, "Compozine inflames the nerves and causes a flareup like this." He told the nurse I was not to get Compozine again and that I would be given another anti-nausea drug as soon as the infusion was over. Again I had the feeling of being a hapless guinea pig, wondering that all drugs used aren't first tested on any patient in minuscule amounts, but the sick weakness of my spinning head and the utter wretchedness of my churning stomach had emptied me of anger and resentment too.

I did not want to look at that pouch with its Chinese-water-torture slow dwindling of liquid. The attacks of vomiting, though just as violent, were intermittent now. I could gulp in air, I could use a handkerchief, and finally, at last, the flow stopped, the final droplet entered the tube, and then the nurse clamped it shut. She tried to comfort me any way she could. As soon as she had taken the intravenous needle out of my wrist and put on a Band-Aid she wiped my face and throat with a cool astringent. "Lie back," she urged, patting my pillows into comfortable shape. Instead, I struggled up. I had to try to stand, to test my legs, see if I could find my equilibrium again, do something, make some move against the awful feeling of loss and woe that pervaded me, the awful consciousness of what was in my body. All I could think of now was that tomorrow Bill was coming to take me home! Away from the hospital, I'd regain some objectivity, make some peace with the fact that in six weeks I must do it all over again. It was best not to think about what was happening inside my body now. Chemotherapy was something I would have to live with if I wanted to live at all, apparently. I put all my hope into the thought of tomorrow, Bill, and home.

When Bill picked me up the next morning I wanted to make a stop before going home. By the time we had gotten checked out and to the car it was almost noon, and I wanted to go to a favorite restaurant. "But aren't you supposed to lose your appetite?" he asked.

"Yes, and it wouldn't do me any good to lose the weight I would lose if I stopped eating. Let's go to Jasper's. I'm going to eat as if I'm ravenous even though I am not."

When an enormous plate of veal piccata and a side dish of spinach had been set in front of me I found that I could will up an appetite. Bill was amazed as I ate, but to me it was basic to my plan. I would enjoy life and the things I had always enjoyed. And I would do everything possible to help with my treatment. I enjoyed Jasper's veal piccata and spinach, and the nutrition they provided would certainly help my treatment.

One of the things I came home to was an international pile of mail. Ever since I'd been told of my cancer, I'd been searching for more information on state-of-the-art cancer treatment in every advanced country. I had written to clinics and research centers asking what they were doing. Surprisingly, I had quite a few answers, but I needed a professional ally to help me understand them. I needed a doctor to guide me through the latest theories and therapies, and I hoped that my internist, a good, compassionate man, would be the one to do the job.

I sat in his office with pad and pencil, listening to the result of my latest examination. His prognosis for me was far more optimistic than Dr. Jaretzki's. (In fact, he dismissed Dr. Jaretzki's six-month prophecy.) Yes, lung cancer had a low survival rate of 4 percent, but my particular kind of adenocarcinoma grew and developed very slowly. With the proper treatment, and my apparent vitality, he thought I had a good chance of reaching the five-year survival plateau, after which one might begin to mention cautiously the word "cured."

"I would like to meet someone who has survived beyond five years," I said. "It would be very helpful."

"Well, there's always Arthur Godfrey."

Godfrey! Columbia Presbyterian's blue-ribbon winner in the survival stakes. But hadn't Dr. Jaretzki assisted at the Godfrey operation? Wasn't that one of the reasons I had gone to him in the first place? And Dr. Jaretzki had expressed no optimism for me!

I asked the question I'd been saving: What if the standard treatments show no improvement in my case? Where else shall I turn? I'd heard of a new immunological therapy called BCG being researched at Sloan-Kettering Institute. Shouldn't that be investigated on my behalf?

Dr. Stock's reaction was negative. Tangentially, he knew of the Sloan-Kettering BCG therapy but he felt that it carried unacceptable risks since the injections involved made use of a live bovine tubercular virus and the danger of contracting TB through the treatment was great.

I thanked him, saying, "This is exactly the sort of information I need from you. I need an objective evaluation of all the facts and data I'm accumulating in my search."

"What search?" The tone was suddenly starchy, even hostile, reminding me of Dr. Jaretzki's reaction. I explained what I had been doing, how the information had accumulated and the fact that I needed help.

"Why do you want to know so much, and above all what good would it do?" the doctor asked.

I sat without answering. There it was again, the professional parochialism, the refusal to consider other approaches that might exist outside a particular doctor's own medical affiliations. This good man was truly upset. So was I, because I knew I couldn't count on him for the special help I needed!

Perhaps he thought I was denigrating my treatment in his hospital, Columbia Presbyterian, but I have never done so. Quite the opposite. I have always been impressed with the quality, personnel, patient care and general facilities at Columbia Presbyterian—but did that mean I should stop searching further to find help for myself? Discoveries were being made in many places, yet the prevailing attitude of the medical staff— and I suspect it's equally true in other large, prestigious institutions—seemed to be that if a new development in cancer research wasn't happening there, it wasn't happening. Of course I couldn't accept that.

The first decision I made concerned the BCG immunological treatment. My quest for information had brought me news of

Israeli research that seemed close to developing the same vaccination but with a chemically synthesized bacillus, much less dangerous than the live one. I would wait to see how that research developed before moving toward BCG, even if my standard treatments failed. Since I had only common sense as a rudder, I'd be doubly wary now, asking more questions about short- and long-term effects before taking any treatment and wanting all possibilities considered for my benefit. I would have to analyze all information on my own, not by choice, and I was very conscious of the perils. But I felt that I had no alternative.

*CHAPTER VII*

# Conventional Medical Treatment

The way to the hospital's sub-basement where radioactive therapy was given led down and down, and as Bill and I followed the arrows pointing through a series of corridors that began on the main floor of Columbia Presbyterian's old building, we were struck by the deepening dinginess of the walls, the musty air of neglect. We wound through a labyrinth of doors, past several waiting rooms filled with dispirited patients, weary or weeping or burdened with tired children. At last the arrow trail ended at a freight elevator. There was one more sign: NUCLEAR THERAPY, 3rd SUB BASEMENT, and an arrow pointing straight down into the depths. The air was heavy with stale cigarette smoke—about three weeks' accumulated stubs uncollected in a sand-filled tub, but there was something else, too; the almost palpable scent of fear, the accumulated dread of the unknown thing in the sub-basement. Suddenly I knew I didn't want Bill to go down there with me. I didn't want him to inhale that dread, that consciousness of radiation burning through human tissue. I didn't want Bill to think of me under the rays.

No, I wanted him to go upstairs, outside, away from here. I asked and he refused, wanting to go with me all the way. I made a hysterical scene right there by the elevator, voice pleading and quavering, angry tears starting, and it finally convinced him that he shouldn't tilt my precarious stability any further.

"Go upstairs. Wait for me in the car. Please, please!" I implored.

"All right, I will if you promise to regain your composure," Bill said.

It was advice I needed. Alone, the creaking freight elevator carried me down and opened on a room vast and dimly lit, empty except for two technicians, a desk and an enormous wheel of file cards. My name was found and I was directed on through two huge protecting doors. Again, I stood in another large empty hall—everything outsize, everything looking like a movie set for Dante's Inferno as directed by Fellini—and heard a voice, floating from some invisible speaker, call my name. "Mrs. McGrail, Mrs. McGrail, go to waiting room number three." All that was missing was the hollow echo.

There were several small waiting rooms and number three was typical: eight chairs, a few magazines on a table and some hauntedly silent people. All of them turned to look at me. I became very conscious of the color in my own cheeks for they had none. Each shared the same waxy pallor; it glistened even in the dim light on the bald skull of a man whose scar showed he'd had an operation for a brain tumor. It was pearly around the horribly bulging eye of a poor little child who was bald from chemotherapy, and it lay across the lackluster expressions of the others. I stood silently accused of health, of appearing there with rosy cheeks and my own hair. Thank God for camouflage, for the will to artifice; I did not want to become like these people, drained of vitality, though they had come to be saved! I thought, I don't belong here, I will never let this happen to me, I don't belong here at all. The others seemed to agree wordlessly.

Again I heard my name on the loudspeakers—no nurses or receptionists down here in the sub-basement—and again I went down a corridor through still another set of huge doors and into one more office space. The chief of radiotherapy was there, the same doctor I'd met at my bedside soon after my operation. She was still cheery, still casually sympathetic.

"Hi there. How are you feeling? You look very well. Shall we take your weight?"

As I weighed in at one hundred and fifteen pounds, I asked her to brief me on anything that might happen during the treatment, any side effects that might become apparent immediately.

"That's hard to say," she answered. "You can expect discoloration of the skin over the first few treatments and there will be a gradual edema. You won't be able to wear anything that presses you closely. And you'll have nausea, but it's a normal reaction."

"What else, Doctor?"

"Your weight. We keep a careful record, because you will be losing fifteen to twenty pounds."

"Will that be due to the nausea?"

"In the beginning. But by the third week of the treatments, you'll find that your esophagus closes and you won't be able to swallow. That's where the major weight loss comes . . . but again, it's a normal reaction to the treatment. After you've finished, you'll have to try very hard to get that weight back."

Surely, I thought, there must be some way around these "normal reactions"!

And I asked, "What if I went on a super-diet of some kind, with a very heavy intake of vitamins and proteins? Wouldn't that help to offset the side effects?"

She shook her head. "Nutrition has no relation to the treatment. Eat whatever you want, whatever you can manage."

"But diet is so important in treating many other diseases."

"Not here, Mrs. McGrail. There is nothing in the world that will minimize these side effects. Nutrition and radiotherapy do not interact."

The doors on the other side of the room opened. A man walked out, slowly, carefully. We did not look at each other.

"The machine is free now."

I followed her into a huge room, fit for a medieval castle and entirely empty, except at its center, where stood a giant X-ray machine painted robin's-egg blue. It was a flash vision of the future—intricate, commanding, nuclear—and we moved toward it respectfully, like acolytes. With very little effort I could imagine the machine as master, its mechanical will served by doctors and patients alike. How else to explain the fact that patients came willingly here, doctors prescribed, technicians administered, all with the same knowledge of how ruinous the therapy was for the human body, how hazardous the cure. People bargained for bits of time—or for years, with luck—by becoming burnt offerings here.

Stripped to the waist, I climbed onto the machine and lay flat on a table which could tilt to accommodate any angle. The X-ray apparatus, a marvel of hydraulically operated precision, could, at the touch of a button, turn, go around, and even go under the table.

As I lay there, the chief radiotherapist outlined a box on my chest with red and black markers; this enclosed the area to be bombarded by rays. Little arrows pinpointed the deepest concentration of rads. "Don't wash anything off," she warned me. The markings insured the technicians' precision, a very vital precaution since any little error could blast a healthy organ with lethal radiation. Tomorrow's radiotherapy session would duplicate this process on my back; I'd collect more red and black "decorations" there.

The technicians dodged back into the glassed-in control

booth from which they operated the machine. I lay waiting, bracing myself, stiff with apprehension, and then . . .

"Sign this, Mrs. McGrail. It's a permission form we need."

A technician had a paper in her hand. I wanted to read it but my glasses were in my handbag across the room.

"Would you read it to me, please?"

She hesitated. When she finally did read it aloud, I understood that reluctance. The permission posed destructive possibilities I hadn't even imagined, naming organs I'd never thought of as involved and disclaiming responsibility for conditions that might occur years from now. It was in fact an absolution for the hospital, freeing it from blame for any ongoing effects of the therapy. It was chilling to hear, but I signed the paper. After all, I had come to obtain those future years for myself. Who wouldn't sign under the pressure of the moment, lying there on that monster machine? I couldn't very well wriggle out from under the cone pointing at my chest and ask to see a lawyer! I was a cancer patient, my life needed saving, I hadn't time.

The beam was positioned over my target area, the machine moved even closer to me, and suddenly the buzzing, whirring noise began. The noise didn't frighten me, the idea of the ray's silent destruction was far more fearsome. My racing imagination set up a silent, mental defense. Against the burning of my tissue and cells, I thought, Water! I imagined deep cooling water flowing over my body. I saw myself splashing in the lake, then swimming in the pounding surf with waves rolling over me. I was deep in water, holding myself there, willing myself an escape from the burning and scorching of my flesh. All the while the machine buzzed on, I was floating deep in icy cool waves and at the end of my treatment, I hardly heard it stop. Then I was shaken gently, helped off the machine, helped into my clothes and I went back to the waiting room.

Bill was there! I was jolted to see him standing outside the door—Bill! And then I was glad, so glad, my hysterical anger forgotten, my idea of sparing him the trauma of the place forgotten, and I reached for him, fell into his arms for a big bear hug. We clung. I needed the support of his arms, the support of his love. He took my hand, we went back to the freight elevator, rode up and followed the path out of the labyrinth, up to the normal world, the sun and air.

It was a bright sunny world outside the hospital, but in a few hours I began to feel sick. There was no pain, only a shivering squeamishness, a light, protesting tremor thrumming through my body, and finally an enveloping nausea that panicked me when I looked at a clock and saw that it was close to lunchtime. Far in advance of this treatment, I had resolved to follow a normal schedule, make as few concessions to it as I could, for I knew that normalcy was a powerful weapon against the ''idea'' of cancer. But it was lunchtime, which to us meant eating at a nearby French restaurant, usually with business contacts. Could I do it? I remembered the day I'd come out of chemotherapy, checking out of the hospital and right into a favorite restaurant; eating, though my ribs stabbed like red-hot knives. I'd smiled, reached for normalcy and found my reward. Today we found a charming small place which served us a beautifully enticing lunch, but the delicacies did no good. This time I couldn't lift the food from my plate. I pushed it about, using the activity to keep down the nausea that was making everything repellent, the nausea threatening to spill out through my nose and ears. Useless—I finally couldn't control it. With teeth tightly clamped together, I nudged Bill urgently and we took leave as gracefully as possible.

Bill put me to bed, making small, kindly, risqué remarks about a noonday bedding. I lay still but it didn't improve and as the hours wore on I wondered about the twenty-four treatments ahead of me. Was this what I had to look forward to tomorrow, the next day and for weeks after that? Life would come to a stop. I hated that idea but I was helpless against it. As I lay there, eyes closed against the endless twisting in my stomach, Bill said, "Suppose there is something we can work out that would prevent this from happening?"

"They told me to expect terrible nausea!" I said.

"Then we'll expect it. But let's reschedule the treatments so that you can have a normal day. Take the treatments late in the afternoon, then we'll come home, you'll go to bed and sleep off the bad effects at the natural time. You'll feel better in the morning and you won't have to face the thing again till the day is almost over. How does that sound?"

It sounded like pure genius. Immediately, I felt a little better. I think the idea of spending my days as an invalid and putting a complete stop to all our activities had depressed me as much as the nausea.

Bill was sweeping on to other grand solutions. "Your stomach's empty. I know you'd feel better if you could eat something."

"Please," I shuddered.

"Oatmeal," said Bill suddenly. "Irish oatmeal, the whole-grain stuff. It's easy enough for a hangover stomach. Suppose I make a big batch now and we have it for breakfast tomorrow?"

At least he didn't expect me to eat it now. I do like Irish oatmeal, but the nausea closed in again. I lay there, not particularly conscious of time or not caring, and then something wonderful happened. Bill was in the kitchen and the rich, grainy smell of the oatmeal he was cooking reached me, twitched at my imagination, somehow slipped past the nausea and suddenly I was tasting it, imagining the warm, nutty texture, the bland, comforting weight in the stomach. I suddenly wanted a bowl of Irish oatmeal. I needed it. I craved it.

"I'll have just a spoonful," I called to Bill.

He brought a porridge bowl full. I ate it all.

Irish oatmeal calmed me out of the stomach knots. Not only was my nausea alleviated but the protesting tremors of my body seemed to quiet. I slept, a whole and quiet sleep. Later, I was to find that Bill's random intuition was right on target: whole-grain oatmeal is considered a nutritional specific for repair of a traumatized nervous system and doctors who do believe in nutritional cancer therapy recommend it to their patients. But all I knew that night was that I could eat it, that something would go down. I promised myself that if necessary I'd live on Irish oatmeal through the whole miserable treatment.

Each day, in spite of my trips to the machine, the nausea lessened. I wanted to share my discoveries with my pale, lethargic fellow patients. Perhaps not many of them could rearrange their schedules to prevent day-long nausea, but all could benefit from the wonderful calmative Irish oatmeal. I couldn't wait to tell the radiotherapist and certainly expected an interested reaction from her, but the way she murmured "Very interesting" indicated sheer indifference. As far as I know, she never mentioned the matter any further. I was baffled then, I'm baffled still by her rejection of the discovery, but I had other things on my mind. Now that I felt better, I wanted to resume a normal life.

We rise early. Bill's up at six, I'm ready to face the world by seven. We love to read our *Times* over fresh orange juice and coffee, play with our two fat city cats and enjoy the early sunlight sparkling through the eastern-exposure windows. None of that changed now. I rose early, was able to add fresh fruit to my oatmeal—bananas always, figs now and then—and make our breakfast interlude the best part of the day. I did make a rule that I followed as soon as breakfast was over: I got dressed—no lingering looks back at the bed. I got dressed and stayed dressed, never slipping back into a bathrobe until bed-time. I wanted no deviation from my normal schedule. Even when I felt miserable—and there were many such moments—I found improvement if I curled up on a living room couch and reached for a book and an afghan.

I didn't want to lose the sense of myself. People complimented me on how well I looked, but I knew that my hair had gone, and my insides were being burned and scrambled. Yet, I felt attractive in spite of everything. Since I hadn't lost weight, my clothes fitted and I thoroughly enjoyed my good fortune. I bought more wigs and Bill kept my perfume in generous supply. The last thing I could bear would be an aura of invalidism. There was an extra special dimension of tenderness between Bill and me these days.

We made plans to entertain again. Entertaining is part of our business life: Bill, a textile and sportswear manufacturer, works with worldwide fashion companies and personalities, makes his New York office in our apartment, and the world comes to us, usually for lunch. Because of my evening radiotherapy sessions, we couldn't take on as large or as frequent luncheon or dinner parties so we settled for a maximum of sixteen business friends at a time for a midweek luncheon and a menu of seasonal specialties that Bill and I, both dedicated cooks, could handle in advance.

Some of our friends and acquaintances couldn't even face the prospect of seeing me, but most were wonderful. I hoped for the best on the day of our first "re-entry" lunch. I spent a long time on the details of it. There was timidity, and some appropriately funereal expressions on our friends' faces. Then quick second looks, then startled relief. It hadn't seemed to me that I'd changed—there was none of the discoloration, none of the swelling I'd been told was inevitable—and now here was confirmation, here was encouragement from others. We sat down around the long Spanish table and I really ate. Food was a pleasure for the first time in weeks! My appetite brought questions about the treatment I was taking, then my first laughter at someone's tentative humor completely lifted what was left of the she-has-cancer pall. Talk around the table turned loose and easy, the lunch was a success. Our friends went away convinced that the McGrails were still active and that business with us could go on as usual.

Taking on more and more of my usual concerns, I found that my energy expanded to fill the need. Mornings were best and happiest, the active middle of the day left no time for anticipation or reflection, and it was not until three in the afternoon that I knew again I was Cinderella with time running out. Then my body began to anticipate the machine, to tremble involuntarily at the knees, go cold in useless protest. I'd take my treatment and after it was over, make my only real concession to cancer by going to bed. Bill, who has always kept farmer's hours, joined me in my early bedtime. We watched the seven o'clock news and went to sleep. Yes, sleep—and without pills for me. I think it was because of my deliberately crowded days, but even the effort of keeping myself as myself, holding on and not giving in, was a daily process that demanded total concentration. I was honestly tired.

After the first week through my radiotherapy I read an article about a Dr. Chereskin in Alabama who reported excellent results in managing the side effects of radiation with a supernutritional diet. His tests involved patients who were undergoing deep radiotherapy and the results in a majority of cases showed that the patients either completely avoided or greatly minimized the things that I had been told were inevitable. Additionally, many of the tumors were completely destroyed.

I went to my own doctors first with the article. But they hadn't heard of Dr. Chereskin, they hadn't heard of his nutritional therapy—and here it was again—they seemed disinclined to follow any purely nutritional lead. I was told again by the radiotherapist that "nutrition and radiotherapy do not interact." So I went home and called Alabama.

Dr. Chereskin was wonderfully accessible. He sent me a

good deal of literature, told me of his own troubles in gaining serious attention from the medical establishment, and on our first call he spent ample time explaining the details of the diet he recommended. I began the next day and immeidately found that it suited me very well.

The rules I followed on the Chereskin diet were these: no processed white sugar, no meat except the white meat of chicken, lots of fresh vegetables, carrots taken raw to obtain the most Vitamin C and Vitamin A, fresh fruit, also eaten raw, fish and eggs. I could use honey as a sugar substitute; its carbohydrates are natural and digestible. And as a first priority, I was to take whole-grain oatmeal every day for its therapeutic effects on the nervous system and its concentrated nutritional value!

Coincidentally, using such quantities of oatmeal, I had already started on the Cereskin diet. It was full of other foods I enjoyed but I needed a doctor's urging to make me eat. Most of the time I still had a monumental disinterest in food. I didn't want to eat but I could, and since I appreciated the distinction, I did. Slowly I became aware that something was happening.

Perhaps I should say that something was not happening. It was well past the dreaded third week and my esophagus had not closed. I ate and maintained my weight. At each session the radiotherapist weighed me carefully; finally she asked questions. I answered fully and freely, described my diet program and saw it noted on my record. But again that seemed to be the end of it. I had a feeling that the doctors classified me as a personal phenomenon with some strain of resistance peculiar to me alone, and not as an experience that could be usefully applied to other patients. Certainly they didn't credit the diet with my success.

But I did credit the diet and I also gave credit to my regime of regular activity, the resolute normalcy of everything we did. Hope, discipline and activity seemed to work together with the selective nutrition. My body was responding, my spirit moving past the first discouragement, all of me opting for survival on my own terms. I felt good, and then it was time for my second chemotherapy treatment.

Since radiation is a killer of white blood cells, a destroyer of natural immunology, and I had had so much radiation, it was necessary now for me to have a blood count to see if it was safe to have chemotherapy again, since chemotherapy also destroys white blood cells. After the first chemotherapy, my blood count had dropped from my normal 5,600 to 2,500, and that was uncomfortably close to the danger point of 1,500, below which no chemotherapy could be given. But a routine examination by the chemotherapist showed that my count had built up to 3,500 in spite of everything and it was considered safe to go ahead. The chemotherapy involved a day's stay in the hospital: checking in before eleven in morning, having the chemicals administered to me sometime during the afternoon and going home the following morning, again before eleven. It was useless to try to prepare myself for it! I was tense and frightened, the nausea returning, not from radiation but from memory of that first chemotherapy session. But I had six more to go, I must take it in stride, I couldn't let my aversion to nitrogen mustard gas dominate me. Hopefully, this time might be easier.

They took the IV needle out at the end of the treatment, and no sooner had they done it than my insides exploded. I staggered to my feet—walking was impossible as violent diarrhea seized and shook me—I hurried toward the bathroom. I slipped, fell and crawled on, but too late, too late. I was stupid with wretched animal misery as I vomited and fouled my clothes. It was worse, ten times worse than before. Even when I was lifted, cleaned up, taken away and put in bed. I had the memory of my guts pouring out of me, and a weak, shuddering sickness that lasted all night and into the morning. I knew Bill was coming at 10 A.M. I meant to be dressed by then but my racked viscera had wrung me dry of strength and energy; I couldn't finish in time.

He gently began to help me dress. He didn't need to ask me how I felt. I volunteered that "the doctor says it will all go away as soon as I get home and rest." Bill nodded without speaking, and with moisture in his eyes.

But at home I did not improve. The weakness lingered. I began to feel feverish and there were intermittent pains in my chest. We called the chemotherapist at his office and asked him what we should do.

"Do nothing," he answered. "These are symptoms of the drug's activity. The pains in the pleural cavity mean that the drug is working there."

I thought that odd. My violent reaction had been to the introduction of the toxic drug and not to its function of killing cancer cells. The chemotherapy hadn't hurt after the treatment the first time. Why should it hurt now?

My illness continued. Two days later my temperature was one hundred and three degrees and the chest pain had sharpened unbearably. My breathing was accompanied by a hollow rumble; breathing itself was becoming difficult. I asked Bill to call the chemotherapist again.

"Never mind that glib charmer. I don't trust him. Let's call Dr. Stock."

I had the problem most patients face in this age of specialization: too many doctors involved. I had the chemotherapist, the radiotherapist, the internist, even the surgeon. Who was "in charge" of my case? I realized that my internist was the overall coordinator; but I thought that since the problem had been caused by chemotherapy I ought to contact the chemotherapist.

Incredibly, he disclaimed the need. But I dragged myself to his office, where he checked my records, took my temperature and assured me that it was normal. He listened to the noises in my chest and said he heard nothing to worry about. My head burned, my chest hurt and my breath rasped, but his casual joviality reduced it to the level of "just nerves." Those were almost the words he used. He said, "This is your imagination working. Go home and rest. Stop worrying. You're just fine."

I walked out of there with a mist before my eyes, part of it weakness, most of it pure fury. I was not "just fine"! For some reason, this doctor was refusing to treat me, refusing to take responsibility. I'd never imagined that such a thing could happen.

Bill and I headed for Dr. Stock's office. When he saw me he made an immediate examination. My temperature registered one hundred and three degrees, just as it had at home. To his ears, the rumble in my chest was pleurisy. And to my surprise he immediately called the chemotherapist and blasted him in my hearing. It was probably a "first" for both these doctors with a patient standing by. I heard Dr. Stock angrily question the chemotherapist. But then, as the conversation lengthened, my internist's expression changed. He calmed, he listened, something else was being discussed.

When he hung up the phone, he said, "This was no way for the chemotherapist to handle today's matter, but . . ."

I waited, wondering what he could say.

"You know we have to take big risks in a case like yours. It's important to find out the limit of your tolerance to drugs. So it's not uncommon early in chemotherapy for the patient to be given a massive dose . . ."

"Do you mean an overdose?"

"It's given intentionally, Mrs. McGrail, as part of the calculated risk of treatment. In your case, this doctor was anxious about the metastic colonies of cancer cells in your pleural area. He had to try to get them, but he had to find out the limit of your tolerance first."

"And this is the result of his experiment, the fever and the pleurisy?" My doctor nodded.

I wasn't mollified. "Why didn't he admit it instead of saying that I was just fine?'' Did he really believe that he could convince me that I was just fine?

Dr. Stock, a paragon of integrity and candor, couldn't understand either, but my question went unanswered. Whatever the medical information gained from that ''calculated risk,'' I was three weeks recovering from the sickness caused by the massive dose, three bedridden weeks during which I could not take any other treatments. I lost strength, I lost ground and I certainly lost patience.

There were questions implicit in the whole method of treatment that I could not solve. I felt comparatively well most of the time, cancer or no, and I became very sick after each treatment. Was I really gaining time for my body or were the combined therapies breaking down my body's natural resistance to such a degree that it would be actually harder for me to fight the disease? If the cure can be as hazardous as the cancer, wasn't it all a Hobson's choice? I couldn't really sort out my attitudes because the stark fact of death kept intruding. Cancer kills. Treatment is mandatory. But are the risks in treatment fully presented to the cancer patient; are they fully taken into account by him? I remembered that Doctor Jaretzki had told me almost casually that with inoperable tumors such as mine, surgery seems to speed the rate of metastasis, adding the authority of his august professional pronouncement to the folk wisdom which says: ''When they cut you open and let the air get at it, it spreads faster.'' But I didn't question just the benefits of surgery. What was radioactive therapy doing besides, one hoped, arresting or shrinking my tumor? How could chemotherapy wrack my body as mercilessly as it did and not also do real damage? And, most basic of all the questions, was it worth the discomforts, the agonies and the effort that the treatments involved to prolong my life if life was to be nothing more than an endless round of treatment?

# CHAPTER VIII

# In Search of Wong Lien

The day I heard of Wong Lien I was in the mood for a miracle. My chemotherapy was almost finished, and while I kept up with all of the treatments and habits conventional medicine prescribed, I wanted to investigate other, perhaps less orthodox, cancer treatments. No treatment I have ever had or heard of has been less orthodox than Wong Lien.

I first heard of Wong Lien through a friend, a food and restaurant editor who was spending a weekend with us. We had not seen each other for some time, so Barbara hadn't known about my having cancer until we started exchanging news of our recent lives. When she heard she wept, but even as she did she began to think of anything she might know that could help me.

What emerged from memory was the story of a man, the brother of a Chinese restaurateur she knew. He was a victim of cancer of the liver who had been given his death sentence, yet had lived. As Barbara recalled it, the man had written a letter of farewell to his mother in Taiwan and had been surprised to receive an urgently practical answer. With the letter came a packet containing a supply of a certain medicinal bark that his mother asked him to brew into tea and drink religiously. Two years after the verdict of doom, his doctors could find no trace of cancer.

"Let's call the Chinese restaurateur," Barbara said. "Perhaps we ought to try him in the morning," I replied. She couldn't wait! "No. Tonight!" Better yet, she'd drive the forty miles to the restaurant, see him, and if possible, get a sample of the miraculous bark. She urged me to come into town early the next morning. "I'll either have some of the stuff or find out where you can get it."

I did. An envelope left for me at our apartment contained a note with the name of the man she had contacted, an address in Chinatown, a list of instructions and something else, something pungently scenting the envelope. I sniffed at a piece of exotically mottled bark shading from vivid yellow to orange to brown. This was "Wong Lien"! I wondered what substances would be released by boiling it into tea: something potent was there, for the note emphatically instructed, "Not to be taken with chemotherapy." But I was taking chemotherapy! Did the instruction mean not to take Wong Lien on the same day as a chemotherapeutical infusion or not to take it at all until the course of treatments was over? I saw that the note contained the address of a special apothecary shop in Chinatown. I was to go there, mention the name of the Chinese friend, and buy a supply of Wong Lien bark. I had the impression that I had best remember that name or no Wong Lien. It must be contraband, I thought, since the whole procedure seemed reminiscent of speakeasy days. Wong Lien must be illegal in this country.

Once that would have disturbed me. But there are too many substances safely used in Europe still awaiting clearance from the Food and Drug Administration here. No, I couldn't wait for bureaucratic clearance, I had cancer! If Wong Lien could help, nothing would stop me. It was raining heavily, but Bill and I decided to go to Chinatown immediately. He got into a raincoat and hat. I bundled in raincoat and scarves. We couldn't wait a minute—I was always in a state of hope but now even Bill's good cool common sense gave way before the idea of a Chinese miracle cure.

The address at first seemed a mistake; it looked less an apothecary's than a front for a bookie joint. The few customers drifting in and out had glazed bettors' eyes; they talked and argued rather than bought, and indeed, there seemed little to buy in the few root- and powder-filled jars on display. The place felt contraband, an impression reinforced by the tall Chinese with pockmarked skin and suspicious eyes who blocked our progress at the door. His English was fluent—at first. We gave the name of our contact, showed our sample of bark, and he seemed to recognize both. "Yes, yes, we have it." As he turned to the drug counter, Bill reached into his breast pocket for my friend's letter—and everything seemed to stop. I can imagine what that startled Chinese saw: a big man with Irish features and official gravity, a big man in a raincoat that could belong to any lieutenant of detectives, a burly six-footer reaching into his pocket for what? Badge? Search warrant? Certainly trouble. At once the shopkeeper—I still think "bookie"—fell back on a time-honored tactic: he misplaced his English. It was "No have, no know" and some fast footwork that moved us backward to the door. In vain, we pointed to what looked like Wong Lien in a jar; we heard "No. No. Mistake please" all over again and then we were standing in the street as the door of the shop clicked shut in our faces.

"Strike one," said Bill; there seemed no point pressing it further. We turned and walked—I don't remember just why— straight across the street into a clean and welcoming Chinese grocery store. The proprietor spoke good English and his attitude was so friendly that we told him our troubles. Wong Lien? Of course he knew it, of course he knew where we could get it. He gave us the number of another shop: the number, rather than the name, since numbers cause less confusion to an outsider. The proprietor came out of his shop to make sure we went in the right direction.

Shop Number Two was the real thing. Through the window we could see rows of shining jars, bins of roots and plants, powders, bottles, salves; a proper place with wizened old people who seemed proper customers. Yet Bill hesitated.

"We blew it before. Perhaps we'd better try to find out something about this place before we go any further. Let's ask around."

The shop we next went into featured gourmet kitchenware in its windows; the gleam of copper drew Bill's eye and in the fit of enthusiasm that usually comes over him in the presence of *implements de cuisine*, he began lifting things off the walls and piling them on the counter. I waited only a moment until he established his status as a serious customer and then began to talk to the proprietor, a lady who spoke fluent British-English.

Wong Lien? Again, there seemed no secret to it. It was very effective and we could certainly buy it across the street. She herself had used it when her daughter was born. In her part of China, all babies received a teaspoon of Wong Lien at birth. She scrutinized me—was I perhaps pregnant? I hurriedly told her my story: my inoperable lung cancer, the tip about Wong Lien. She began to hedge a bit in her enthusiasm; I should have seen and evaluated that. Well, she continued, it was true that Wong Lien was marvelously effective in many conditions, but she thought I ought to see the doctor in the apothecary store for the use that I intended to make of it.

"Is there a doctor there?" I was surprised.

Yes, there was a Chinese doctor and I ought to get advice on blends and combinations of Wong Lien with perhaps other substances. Our kind lady's capacity to help was exhausted, and so Bill paid for his purchases and we went across the street. Our circuitous route to Wong Lien had been well worth it; obviously, since so many Chinese knew of it and I could speak to a doctor about it, Wong Lien was not illegal: it was accepted, appropriate, potent, perhaps a miracle for me after all!

And there it was in the apothecary's, a whole weird, mottled bin of it, selling for a relatively reasonable seventeen dollars per ounce. As we bought an ounce, I asked for an appointment with the doctor. The man behind the counter seemed puzzled, but motioned me toward his rear door. I left Bill waiting in the front of the shop and went through the rear door alone.

It opened into a small vestibule. The corridor was lined with benches where people sat knee-to-knee; the doctor's office was a makeshift cubicle partitioned off from the "waiting room" and curtained at its entrance; certainly there was not enough room to swing open a door either way. Sibilant conversation among the seated Chinese at my entrance alerted the doctor: she came out to see me and I looked down at her, from my full height of five foot four inches. She was as frail as a bird whose outline is suggested in a few artistic Chinese brush strokes, oddly girlish, certainly nonmedical. But in her "office"—a desk, a chair, and a bed covered with the shoe marks of previous patients—I did see what was obviously a Chinese medical diploma.

"You seem so young to be a doctor," I ventured.

She smiled. Had I insulted her? No, the bright eyes, the birdlike voice showed only interest, and though she spoke no further, I went on to tell her my entire medical history. It took a while and still she did not speak, but she nodded occasionally and waited for me to go on. When I had finished, while I was waiting for a comment or a reaction or some advice, she spoke again. "Tomorrow. Come tomorrow at two o'clock."

Why tomorrow? I was here now and I had bought the Wong Lien.

"I'd like to start taking the tea," I told her. "Perhaps you could tell me something about how Wong Lien works?"

"Please come tomorrow at two o'clock."

My time was over. I went out, wondering at our one-sided interview. Perhaps I had barged in, perhaps displaced another patient. Perhaps she wanted to think about my case overnight. Perhaps—what? If only I could discuss Wong Lien with my own internist, but of course he would not have heard of it. I consoled myself with the idea of centuries of Oriental wisdom untapped by Western medicine and so many of our own cures owing their origins to Chinese herbal lore. I was off the beaten track, after all, in this strange little place, but wasn't the odd chance exactly what I was investigating? And I did have an appointment tomorrow at two o'clock.

The next day Bill came into the small corridor with me, extinguishing all extra space and looking around with surprise and apprehension. When I went into the doctor's cubicle, he positioned himself on the other side of the partition, with his ear close to it, an intentional eavesdropper.

I smiled at the doctor. She knew my whole story now, it would help our rapport. And today, of course, she'd do the talking.

I was wrong about that.

"Well?" said the doctor.

I felt a bolt of apprehension.

"You want acupuncture?" she sang out.

Acupuncture? She had never mentioned it. Looking into her bright eyes, I had the feeling that she didn't even remember who I was.

"I'm Mrs. McGrail, I was here yesterday, I have cancer, I want to take Wong Lien, don't you remember?"

She cocked her head, more birdlike than ever, and trilled, "What hurt you?"

I heard Bill get to his feet as the doctor, looking at me again, made another estimate. In a surprisingly loud sing-song she asked, "You going to have baby?"

Bill pushed back the curtain and came in. "My God," he exclaimed, "she doesn't understand English!"

I realized this some moments ago. As we stood together, the doctor made the obvious connection between us and turned to Bill. "What hurt your wife?" she sang out once again.

"Come on, Joie," Bill said sternly. "Let's get out of here."

"Wait," I begged. "There may be something we can learn." As if the doctor had read my mind, she bridged the language gap by reaching for a Chinese-English dictionary, flipping it open to the section with English words and Chinese definitions.

"Here. Show me what wrong with you."

Out of curiosity, I stopped at the C's and pointed to "cancer."

The doctor let out a wail of distress. "No, no. No." Her vocie went louder, keening, higher still: "Can't help; nobody help!"

She looked at me earnestly. I nodded. We went out quietly, followed by head-shaking, tongue-clucking and sounds of compassion from the waiting Chinese. Our interview was public property, and the doctor's farewell was a wide and sweeping gesture of despair.

On the street, laughter overtook us, helpless shaking laughter at the absurdity of it and our own childish gullibility. A tidal wave of laughter washed us down the street, falling against buildings and lampposts, carrying away the accumulated tension. When we stopped, when we got our breath back, we found ourselves in front of a restaurant.

"No miracle cure," said Bill. "How about a miraculous lunch?"

Over lunch, which was indeed very good, we decided that perhaps Wong Lien might have some therapeutical value and we should have the bark analyzed at the Brooklyn Botanical Gardens. Bill and I never put off spur-of-the-moment decisions, so we went right out to Brooklyn to see the curator. He told us that we were fortunate in that a Chinese botanist was in charge of the Gardens and would probably be able to determine the properties of Wong Lien. We shaved off a few snippets of the bark and left it for the Chinese expert. Later, he called to tell us that he couldn't analyze it, and he promised to send the sample to the Harvard Medical School and to Washington, D.C., if necessary. While we waited for an answer, I decided that I had better declare myself to my internist, Doctor Stock, before I brewed and drank Wong Lien tea.

Perhaps of all the surprises of the last few days, Doctor Stock's reaction was the most unexpected. He did not laugh at me. This very distinguished physician and proper Yale man simply said, "I'd like to have it analyzed to be sure that it isn't poisonous to your condition. Otherwise, I don't see how a cup of tea twice a week would do any harm."

In a way, Dr. Stock's reaction deflated my expectations for Wong Lien even further. Doctors have one of two reactions when you suggest stepping off the straight and narrow medical way into speculative treatment: they're either seriously alarmed at what you plan to do or amused at your folly. Dr. Stock's reaction was neither. Still, another bit of Wong Lien bark was sent to Cornell Laboratories, at Dr. Stock's request, and still another group of experts was essentially baffled, saying only that it was nonpoisonous. The Chinese botanist called in to report the same results from Harvard and Washington. So Wong Lien remained an enigma; if it worked in the ways that the ordinary Chinese people used it, no one could say why.

We were never able to connect the bark to cancer except in our friend's hopeful story—the one which had started the entire search. It may have been, in fact it almost definitely was—a chimera we had been chasing. It was our flirtation with a miracle.

We didn't find a cure for cancer, but we did come up with some beautiful copper pots, the satisfaction of mystifying the medical and botanical experts and the pleasure of laughing together at our quest. In times such as we had been having, the laughter alone was worth the effort.

# CHAPTER IX

# Piecing Together
# a Cancer Diet

In September of 1974, as my radiotherapy was ending, I began to think about what I could do in my own behalf. The answer seemed obvious. Special nutrition had spared me the drastic weight loss and other traumas that usually accompany radiotherapy. Now I decided to continue to investigate other ways in which special nutrition could benefit a cancer patient.

It's a wonder I hadn't turned to nutritional therapy sooner. Most people are doctor-and-medicine-oriented: I am not. All my life I have relied on fresh, natural food, reaching instinctively for whatever my body demanded for health at the time. After my cancer surgery, when everything in our country vegetable garden was ripe and ready, I had cravings for more than the dewy fresh peas, young carrots and fingerling zucchini I usually enjoyed. I began to eat greens, snipping off fresh herbs, tasting leaves. During my radiotherapy I was on a steady daily diet of tarragon, sage, fennel, basil, anise, parsley, dill, sorrel—as many as a dozen fresh herbs daily. "You're grazing!" Bill told me. And truly, nothing green was safe from me. I was also drinking pots of Moroccan-style peppermint tea: handfuls of fresh mint stuffed into a large tea glass over which I poured hot mint-brewed tea and added a spoonful of honey. The tea was my champagne, and I seemed to need it every day. Later, when I read the works of the doctor who developed a nutritional therapy for cancer, I found out why I had the craving for fresh greenery. But all I knew then was that I wanted and craved those things. I drank endless pots of peppermint tea, "grazed" faithfully through the garden and continued to take my long-standing health recipe of a clove of garlic, apple seeds and honey every day. I have always believed in the positive good of these things, in the efficacy of natural folk medicine that I took myself and dispensed to my family. The hot milk and honey I gave Bill actually helped rid him of insomnia. I, the cancer patient, fell fast asleep on my milk and honey each night while Bill sometimes fretted sleepless until he tried this old, old remedy. The cures of my childhood guarded our children's health for years. I gave them hot milk with minced garlic and a big dollop of butter for colds and/or fevers, made them eat half a fresh lemon to unblock a stuffed nose.

My attitude toward "natural" cures was that they were innocent medicine, and I had no notion of the devastating biochemical power that certain combinations of natural foods can have on the human body until I began investigating nutritional therapies for cancer.

I did not come on any information about these therapies through my regular doctors because the medical profession is uninterested in the nutritional aspects of cancer. But one day I found a book that contained fifty cases, documented with before-and-after X-rays, of patients who had been cured of inoperable cancers by a very strict, radical dietary regime. The doctor who had developed the diet and written the book, Dr. Max Gerson, had demonstrated evidence of his cures to the Pepper-

Neeley congressional subcommittee on cancer, bringing with him five patients who had been cured of cancer and the records of all the others. I wondered what had become of Dr. Gerson's method and why, if it could produce cures, it was not in widespread use today.

Dr. Max Gerson first came to international attention in his native Germany in 1929, when his unusual treatment for lupus, a supposedly incurable tuberculosis of the skin, had successful results in 446 out of 450 cases. Dr. Albert Schweitzer, hearing of it, brought his own wife to Dr. Gerson to be cured of tuberculosis of the lungs, and when Dr. Gerson was successful, Dr. Schweitzer declared, "A genius walks among us!" From 1929 to 1933, Dr. Gerson lectured widely in Europe. In 1936, he emigrated to the United States, broadened the scope of his research and devoted himself to chronic degenerative diseases, especially cancer. The Gerson therapy was based on biochemical reactions to certain combinations of natural foods and it was extremely rigorous, requiring constant supervision and regular follow-ups by a physician. The ideal place to take the therapy would have been in Dr. Gerson's clinic, but he had died of pneumonia at the age of seventy-seven in 1959. The clinic no longer existed, the disciples were scattered, and even Dr. Gerson, writing for the future in his book *A Cancer Therapy*, assumed that the physicians reading it would be unfamiliar with his treatment. As a warning to other doctors, he noted, "This is a medical treatment which should be applied by a physician only after thorough examination and correctly adapted to each patient's needs." There was certainly no thought that one day a would-be patient would try to cure herself by the book!

After being told so frequently by my own doctors that "diet makes no difference in cancer," I could scarcely present the book to them, scarcely walk into a medical office and say,

"Cure me by following this." I decided to give it a try on my own. I think the reason was the two seductive words "natural healing." Hadn't I always believed in it? I remembered the German naturopath who had relieved me of the arthritis pain in my right knee at age twenty-two—and done it on a three-month regimen of exactly so many glasses of buttermilk per day, exactly so many glasses of orange juice and precisely three hours of daily exposure to sunlight. The pain, banished thirty years ago, had never returned. That didn't particularly surprise me. I'd had confidence in the intrinsic value of "natural" treatment and I was still using buttermilk as a panacea for nerves and fatigue on the day of my mysterious "heart attack" in the Washington airport. There was, no doubt, hubris in my brave confidence in my ability to follow a natural healing regime on my own. I read Dr. Gerson's *A Cancer Therapy* slowly and carefully, determined to do it myself.

Some of Dr. Gerson's concepts were completely new to me. He saw cancer not as a tumor developing in one or more organs of the body but as a total, degenerative disease resulting from a disfunctioning metabolism. A normal body has reserves to suppress malignancy, he points out, yet in cancer patients the malignancy has grown freely from the smallest cellular unit without encountering suppression. Why? Gerson's answer was that the cancerous body's general immunological systems have become inactivated, poisoned by the fermentative growth of neoplastic cancer cells, quite different in their makeup from the normal cells of the body. He made a clear distinction between noncancerous cells, deriving their energy through oxidation, and cancerous cells, more primitive, energizing themselves primarily through the process of fermentation. Patients with growing cancers fall deeper and deeper into the fermentative process, the bodily balance is tipped against oxidation, and finally the liver, where most metabolic processes are concentrated, is totally poisoned by the accumulated toxins and fails in its functions. When the liver deteriorates and the metabolic balance is upset, the body's natural defense system becomes ineffective and the body can no longer fight the spread of cancer.

Dr. Gerson took issue with the standard cancer treatments. He felt that surgery could certainly bring relief to the body by removal of tumorous masses but that the benefits would be short-lived because surgery cannot solve the problem of the toxification of the liver. He questioned the efficacy of radiotherapy and chemotherapy, doubting the wisdom of attacking a body already in a weakened condition with powerful X-rays, radium and cobalt in a way which damages other parts of the body as well as the tumor site and further hinders its powers to heal itself. He tried to help the body detoxify itself with special medication and special nutrition so that the metabolic enzymes might resume oxidation and restore its lost balance. The body that has endured chemotherapy and radiotherapy successfully is still left with masses of dead toxic cancer cells that must somehow be eliminated. Unless this is done, the tumor—a symptom of the total cancerous condition—will reappear at some other site. To achieve a true cancer cure, Dr. Gerson's therapy had these objectives:

The body must be completely detoxified.

The body must be continuously supplied with ionized minerals and foods with high natural oxidative action so that the essential enzymes can be stimulated into resuming the natural oxidation process.

When the general metabolism is gradually corrected and harmony restored, then the defense immunity system, in which no abnormal cell can develop or grow, is reactivated.

A step-by-step progress toward cure depends on the healing power of the entire body, the total organism.

Of course I identified with the reasoning and objectives of the Gerson therapy. My tumor, inoperable, was still in my body and the mass of it had been attacked by radiotherapy and chemotherapy. The tumor had been killed; of course there would still be an overload of toxic dead cancer cells in my system. If I could eliminate them, if I could consciously help my body to heal itself, I would begin the Gerson therapy at once. I would buy the special equipment needed to prepare the foods and subordinate my living to its schedule. But my first problem would be the medications that accompanied the diet daily. They were detoxified iodine, called Lugol's solution, niacin, thiamine, thyroid grains and, above all, the large quantities of potassium needed first to balance and then to stimulate the metabolic processes. The medications could not be bypassed. Neither the dietary regime nor the medication is effective alone, Dr. Gerson had written. The combination is essential for success.

How was a do-it-yourself patient to determine safe dosages for medications and how to get the necessary prescriptions for them? I had to establish a kind of arm's-length relationship with a naturopath to accomplish it. He knew of Gerson's therapy and prescribed the safe dosages of what were obviously body-building vitamin supplements. I told Dr. Stock about my diet, but he didn't believe it would make any difference in the long run. He felt I'd done all that could be done by completing my radiotherapy and chemotherapy. I'm sure that he considered all my experiments and ''tinkering'' to help myself as stubbornness, a bull-headed refusal to accept the facts.

Everything about the Gerson diet was uncompromising. Pressure cookers or steamers could not be used to prepare the vegetables. A special press was needed. Liquefiers, centrifuges, anything that pierced the skin of the fruit could not be used to make the juices. Another press was needed. No aluminum utensil could be used: I bought only enamel. I bought a food mill to make the special vegetable soup that was a daily diet staple. And I learned that the vegetables and fruits in my supermarket were strictly off limits: nothing sprayed, nothing colored for appearance or preservation, nothing packed in plastic bags could be used. I made arrangements for a continuous supply of organically grown vegetables.

Every item of the Gerson dietary regime was related in its purpose: to detoxify the liver quickly, to supply the body with high-oxidation juices that would stimulate enzyme action, and since potassium is inactive in a cancerous body, to refill the tissues with the all-important potassium. Potassium was supremely important. Sodium extremely dangerous. Dr. Gerson maintained that potassium and its K-group minerals ionized what the body needed with positive electrical potential and kept all processes normal, while sodium and minerals of the sodium group, increasing radically in an absence of potassium, ionized on a negative potential, allowing abnormal processes to develop.

It was something of a race, I found, to keep a sick body filled with what it needed to build health: to fill the tissues with as much potassium as possible, exclude as much sodium as possible, and keep that constant supply of freshly squeezed juices with their short-lived high oxidation coming into the system. The special soup on the Gerson diet could be made up in the morning and used throughout the day, but everything else had to be pressed out on the spot and taken immediately in order to be effective. There were green-leaf juices—what I'd taken in my instinctive "grazing"—to be prepared hourly: lettuce, beet tops, Swiss chard, red cabbage leaves, escarole, endive, romaine, green pepper, watercress. Another constant was the freshly pressed juice of calf's liver, mixed with carrot juice for palatability and taken three times a day to provide the fastest restoration for the human liver. There were three meals, consisting only of vegetables and fruits, to be prepared. Absolutely salt-free. And for still faster detoxification, enemas several times daily: coffee enemas, camomile enemas, green-leaf-juice enemas. (I must confess I bypassed the enemas. My own system of elimination has always been adequate. And with all the extra stimulus of so much fruit and vegetable juice throughout the day, I didn't see how anything further could possibly be necessary.) My crash course in survival, the Gerson dietary regime, took one-third of my waking day: cooking, grinding, pressing, preparing, eliminating, taking medicine.

The list of forbidden foods was animal fats, stimulants, oils, junk food, fermentative foods such as cheese, wine, pineapple, white bread, salt. Strictly forbidden was anything with a high sodium count. That excluded processed, canned and even frozen foods; all contained surprisingly high levels of sodium and preservatives. There was no meat or fish permitted at all, with the exception of the calf's liver juice. Herbs and fruit could be used as seasoning to vary the taste of the dull menu. Vegetables had to be thoroughly washed, had to be unpeeled, and were to be cooked very slowly and without water or salt, though stock of the special soup could be substituted. The Gerson diet allowed switching the order of food intake, but not departure from the regimen because all combinations of food had been selected quite deliberately for their biochemical reactions and importance to the other parts of the total therapy. Dr. Gerson had had his dietary regime evaluated by some of the greatest authorities of his day, such as the famous nutritional biologist, Professor Abderhalden. He had taken advice, closed all loopholes, left nothing to chance. I found it exhaustive—and exhausting.

I am a natural list maker, but my usual "little list" was completely inadequate to remind myself of what foods must be taken. I needed a chart to get through each Gerson day and I made one. A typical day's entry looked like this:

8:30 BREAKFAST
One glass of fresh fruit juice
Large portion of natural Irish oatmeal. No butter, no milk, but honey or stewed fruit might substitute for milk on the oatmeal. A serving of special dark rye saltless bread, toasted or plain. This was the only bread the diet allowed.

9:00 One or more glasses of green juice.

10:00 One or more glasses of fruit juice.

11:00 One or more glasses of fresh carrot and apple juice. The medications: potassium, niacin, or thyroid tablets might be taken with juice. Lugol's solution could also be taken, but not with green leaf juice.

11:30 Liver juice. No medication.

12:30 LUNCHEON
Raw salad of green leaf vegetables.
1 warm glass of special soup. Contents: celery knob, bunch celery, 2 leeks, 1 lb. potatoes, 2 lbs. tomatoes, 2 onions.
1 glass of juice (fruit)
1 large baked potato (or occasional brown rice)
Cooked vegetables
Dessert of raw or stewed fruit

3:00 Liver juice. No medication.

4:30 Liver juice. No medication.

5:00   One or more glasses of green juice.

5:30   One or more glasses of juice.

6:00   One or more glasses of fresh fruit juice. Medication could be
       taken with the juices.

6:30   DINNER
       Raw salad
       1 glass of warm soup
       Large baked potato
       2 cooked vegetables
       Dessert of raw or stewed fruit.

Dr. Gerson added, "Don't drink water. The stomach is needed
for juices and soups."

At first it seemed impossible to eat it all. But, as Dr. Gerson
noted, the food was low in calories, asked little of the metabolism and was quickly digested. It was not a strengthening diet. I
missed protein, I felt weak and irritable, but I was startled to
find that the doctor considered those feelings as normal symptoms of detoxification under way. His book said that in a month
the metabolism should improve, the appetite increase and the
patient could have more of the same food whenever wanted,
even during the night when awake. By that time, I would have
reached the second stage of recovery and might have to adapt
my diet to the "flare-ups" and allergic reactions that were
"further barometers of healing."

But after a month on the Gerson diet, I realized that I was in
well over my head. Dr. Gerson's clinic must have been the ideal
atmosphere for his therapy, not only because the professional
care would relieve you of the constant problems of shopping
and provisioning, but because of the predicted complexities that
would accompany the course of the cure. Dr. Gerson en-

visioned planned allergic reactions as part of his therapy. He wrote that a cancerous body was too weak to develop them and he was trying to reactivate allergic reactions as part of the body's own normal defense network. Gerson patients could develop a variety of predictable reactions: hypersensitivity to sunlight, to any kind of physical or mental exertion, to any form of antibiotic, to the very liver juice or vegetable juice or orange juice on the diet. The doctor corrected nutritional allergies by adding large doses of potassium and adjusting the medication to the problem, but I could not. I was solely responsible for what happened to me. As I went along, the drawbacks to the doctor-less, do-it-myself treatment multiplied. And Dr. Gerson regarded eighteen months on his diet as the minimal time for success!

One day I looked at Bill pressing out a glass of liver juice and thought, Enough! We must stop this! I knew he had become an uncomplaining martyr to my cure. Ironically, I have always loved raw fruits and vegetables, looked forward to eating them, but now that we were knee-deep, covered with celery knobs and cabbage and carrots and apples, the daily treadmill of preparation, ingestion and preparation again had become deadly. Life à la Gerson suddenly demanded too many sacrifices of the people I loved best, destroyed too much of the atmosphere of normalcy I had battled so hard to achieve. This treadmill of survival was life too dearly bought and I could not continue it, even if I did not survive. Every moment of my life with Bill and my family was precious to me and at the rate we were going all we could look forward to at the end of the year was my consumption of 1,000 pounds of carrots, 1,300 pounds of apples, 350 to 450 pounds of liver for juice, 45 heads of lettuce, 70 bushels of celery knobs, Lord-knows-how much red cabbage, 55 bunches of celery, masses and masses of green peppers, and green leaves, green leaves— "Bill," I called suddenly. "Let's call it quits!'' "You're sure?'' he asked. I nodded. My husband smiled in a way that I'd almost forgotten.

Ironically, and this made my defection from the diet difficult, I still believed that Dr. Gerson was correct. His cumbersome and constant feeding was like the first exploration in any new field. If the doctor had lived, he might have found a way to simplify his therapy, make it work for people with jobs and families, make it at least adaptable to normal life. And the list of remarkable cancer cures would have lengthened long past the fifty he documented. But Dr. Gerson was gone and I could not follow his legacy. I gave up the Gerson therapy after a month, still believing in its direction, but aware that I myself could not follow it.

Yet, because of Gerson, I have found it easier to understand and put together the diet I now follow. And I have developed an awesome respect for the biochemical power of food as medicine. Through Gerson's therapy, I've learned that seemingly innocent combinations of food can produce the vilest effects of chemotherapy: uncontrollable vomiting, hepatic coma, a foul, necrotic odor produced by dead cancer cells, an odor I was beginning to be aware of as a general mustiness, but one which became so powerful in the advanced therapy that it blistered the paint in the rooms where Doctor Gerson's patients lay.

And because of Dr. Gerson, I am ever conscious of what I eat. He traced cancer back to the manner in which food is grown and saw chemical interference with it at any level as evil and irresponsible. He warned of the hidden disguises of sodium in diet, the dangers of a sodium buildup. I have stopped eating many foods simply because I know that sodium chloride is used to pickle and preserve, as a heat transfer and blanching agent in frozen foods, as a form of bicarbonate in canning to prevent the toughening of vegetables. (I avoid bicarbonate, both in the popular stomach medications and in the suspiciously green peas and asparagus often served by restaurants. They add a pinch of bicarb to "dress up" the dish.) Sodium propionate is used to inhibit mold. A form of sodium acid phosphate stabilizes evaporated milk and quickens quick-cooking farina. Another form is used to sulfur fruit before it is dried. Saltine crackers never cross my lips, and I carefully avoid a whole host of disguised foods right out of chemical laboratories. I try to protect myself from chemical additives by keeping the Gerson research in mind. I have been able to devise a more livable lifetime diet based on the principles of a man who shared many of Dr. Gerson's ideas, another nutritional innovator, Dr. Ernest Freund.

The Freund diet was advanced in Austria in 1934, gained many adherents and is still well known and widely used in Austria and Germany. Dr. Freund's regime resembles Gerson's in several ways, but it is a far less rigorous diet that does not rule out the possibilities of a normal life or a meal in a restaurant. The Freund diet is a nutritional cancer therapy that can easily be maintained as a lifetime regime.

Dr. Freund made his nutritional breakthrough when he discovered that the serum of cancer-free people and animals contained chemical substances able to dissolve cancer cells. The Freund-Kaminer research team worked for thirteen years discovering that cancer patients' blood not only did not produce this saving substance but actually produced a chemical that was cancer-protective. On the other hand, cancer creates its own optimum environment. And as cancer cells grow and spread, they widen this shield of protective environment until the body's entire balance is tipped toward cancer and against efforts to cure it.

Dr. Freund, like Dr. Gerson, considered cancer a total, degenerative disease rather than a localized condition. The

Freund and Gerson approaches to treatment sounded similar: a thorough cleansing of the body and stimulation of elimination. Freund found that cancer patients had an abnormal amount of fatty acids in their bodies and his angle of attack was to eliminate animal fats from the diet entirely, replacing them with certain less complex vegetable oils. He believed in the struggle between normal cells and fermentative cancer cells, and eliminated all fermentative foods and restricted carbohydrates very sharply. There was one major nutritional disagreement: cabbage. Gerson gave it the highest priority on his regime, Freund eliminated it completely. As I've never liked cabbage, I was happy to follow Freund's dictum, though I wondered how he had achieved any cancer cures among the German and Austrian peasants who were his patients.

Olive oil was forbidden, but I was able to use apricot or almond oil as a dressing for salad. Dr. Freund's diet allowed yogurt, cultured buttermilk and pot cheese. I could continue to take my private recipe of a clove of garlic, apple seeds and honey daily. And I could add wheat germ, a longevity tip from Dr. Szent-Gyorgy, the eighty-four-year-old cancer researcher. This was really *my* diet, following Dr. Freund's general directive, yet combining some of the best features of Chereskin and Gerson. It is a synthesis, a good-sense moderate diet, and a nutritional therapy that I firmly believe is the correct one for me.

## PROHIBITED FOODS

These are the foods I must always avoid: alcohol, bread and yeast products, white sugar, enriched white flour, whole milk and rich cheese, animal fats (including butter), carbohydrates, chocolates, junk food, anything commercially canned, frozen or bottled, artificial coloring or preservatives, oleomargarine, olive oil and coconut oil, pork, ham, or any other fat meat, beef, pineapple, gaseous vegetables, heavy seasonings and spices.

## REQUIRED FOODS

I must eat the following each day:

Fresh orange juice
Irish oatmeal or wheat germ
Honey—at least 1 tablespoon
Banana or fresh figs or dates
2 other fresh fruits
2 raw vegetables (except cucumbers)
1 portion chicken, fish or lean meat
Beet soup with fresh dill (or beet juice, no preservatives)
Yogurt
Buttermilk
1 clove garlic
2 cooked vegetables
Herb tea (fresh mint when in season)

## PERMITTED FOODS

I may eat the following if I choose: whole-grain cooked cereals, pot cheese, occasional eggs (never yolks alone), occasional pasta (made of pure semolina, never of refined white flour), soups of all kinds (vegetable stock base), skimmed milk, dried fruits (unsulfured) and, of course, all fresh fruits and vegetables (excepting the few on prohibited list).

I find this diet flexible enough to adjust to a schedule that takes me out occasionally. And since the protein allowance can be eaten at lunch or dinner, it's possible to have a reasonably satisfactory meal in a restaurant. I often do, sitting far away from the tempting bread and rolls. I don't really think about the forbidden foods; I concentrate instead, since I like to cook as well as eat, on the delicious recipes I can create from the permitted foods on my diet. My favorites: beet soup with dill; Bulgar soup—a robust combination of buttermilk, yogurt, garlic, nuts and dill, from Bulgaria, a land where one hundred years is considered a ripe but not uncommon age; a rose-petal conserve I've made from the flowers in our country garden; moules marinière without butter or wine; fingerling zucchini with an equal volume of fresh herbs (6!); garden sorrel soup; blue fish with mounds of chopped parsley and basil, and pasta al pesto, the irresistible basil pasta of Genoa. By buying the imported Italian pure semolina pasta all worry about refined white flour is eliminated.

I am faithful to my diet without strain. I could not remain on Dr. Gerson's regime for the eighteen months he regarded as minimal for a cure, but I can easily maintain the regime of Dr. Freund. And since it is a "forever" diet, it does allow small treats from time to time. I believe in the positive power of nutritional therapy for cancer. Perhaps the long-sought cure for cancer will be found in nature's storehouse of medications after all.

## CHAPTER X

# Celebrating Too Soon

Of the six months that I had been given to live, five were already gone. But only the calendar said so: my physical condition had improved steadily and I felt better every day. My good health seemed to be real, not just a merciful illusion. My weight was stable at 115 pounds, EKG normal, blood pressure 110 over 70, lungs clear. Blood analysis, urinalysis, kidney function, liver scan—all clear, no sign of cancer. As Doctor Stock kept taking tests, he moved from a noncommittal detachment to cautious elation to medical exuberance. Remission! I was in remission only five months after the morning Dr. Jaretzki had told me to make my will.

The odds against my survival were very high. But apparently the one predictable thing about cancer is that it isn't predictable, and Dr. Jaretzki had said as much when he dropped in on me at Harkness Pavilion before one of the periodic chemotherapy sessions. Luckily, he came before the infusion, when I was glowing with health. Afterward, I'd be quite sick, though not as cataclysmically as in the beginning, and I didn't want anyone to see me then. Dr. Jaretzki said, "You are unusual. You have made a conspicuous recovery." And he added, "Your skin is unbelievable for a cancer patient.'' I remembered our earlier dialogue during which I'd asked if there was anything I could do to help myself and he'd answered, ''Nothing at all.'' Now I was sure that I was where I was because I'd been making positive efforts to fight. And, deep inside, a certainty was growing that I'd achieve a complete cure. The odds against me had been high and somehow I'd managed to hurdle them. So when Dr. Stock said ''remission'' I heard ''rebirth.''

Bill said, ''Let's go to the Caribbean and celebrate in the sun.'' I thought at once of Dick and Stephanie in San Juan. They'd suffered with me from the very beginning; now I could bring them the gift of my deliverance. And we loved San Juan! Bill and I are creatures of habit, preferring to return to loved, familiar places, and to go about the calm routine of other winter vacations spent in San Juan with nothing hanging over us would be absolute happiness indeed. Now I wanted to sink into time without thought. Someone once wrote that the true test of happiness is not knowing what day of the week it is, something a miserable person is aware of even in his sleep. I had been measuring the time I had left to live and now I didn't want to know the difference between Monday and Saturday. We'd throw away the clock, sink into the calm of the tropics where the middle of the day seems to stand absolutely still.

We overpacked, of course. There were so many possibilities to be slowly and peacefully explored and the one all-purpose weekend pants outfit has never been my way to go. But I wasn't prepared for the mountain of luggage we finally took to the airport and I could sympathize absolutely with the expression on Stephanie's face as it filled her front hall. Dick laughed and laughed—it was a souvenir of my days as a fashion editor. Dick considered this absolute proof that I was back to normal. ''Even if you change twice a day every day, some of those bags are going back to New York unopened,'' Dick told me. And he was right.

Dick and Stephanie's house has always reminded me of a choice, small hotel with its twenty-foot beamed ceilings, central patio, marble halls and separate guest quarters on the second floor. Here in old San Juan, love and patience have restored the ambiance of the past. Looking down from our terrace at the steep stairways of old San Juan, we could see the ways that we would take tomorrow; how we would stroll up to El Convento for our second breakfast, where we would find the flower seller, which way to the shops I loved to browse in. Familiar as all these things were, I felt I was seeing them with new eyes. It was part of my recovery, part of my incredible rebirth.

Just the morning sunlight, just the floating armoa of coffee, just the deep azure of the blue-bricked streets—"blue souls" we called those bricks—these things were enough to make me want to cry. It was so sweet, so joyful to be reborn. We ate Stephanie's good breakfast with every intention of eating again—amid the gardenias and lilies in the garden of El Convento, taking coffee with good, nourishing breaths of the sun, the air and the flowers. We do make a thing of flowers, Bill and I. We live for the blooming season of our gardens at home and with all the flowers around us in the plazas, we still couldn't get enough, and had to buy armfuls of tuberoses and torch ginger from the flower seller and bring them back to fill every vase in the house.

Something strange happened on that first day as we strolled the azure street bricks. I tripped and fell. I never recall just falling, and if I did, I would land on balance like my cats, supported on my hands and knees. But this time I sprawled. We checked the surface and found a brick that protruded slightly above the rest, hardly enough to catch my foot. It was unpleasant, not because of the harmless fall, but because it reminded me of the so recent time before my recovery, the dizziness after chemotherapy, the instability I had felt when I had been out of my own control. I shook off the shivers. Nothing must spoil our perfect vacation!

Any happy time is a stringing together of odd little moments, like jewels of pure pleasure on a chain. I remember the evening of the day I fell on the bricks, an evening spent at a fine French restaurant, where we told Dick and Stephanie that I had been given every encouragement for a complete cure. I remember swinging through the night street arms linked, four abreast, nothing wrong with my balance then. And I remember sitting for hours every evening on our terrace until the gentle evening showers drove us inside. I remember love every day, I remember constant happiness with Bill and with Dick and Stephanie . . . and I do remember feeding the cats.

Bill and I feed them every winter; the strays of old San Juan are our scruffy friends. How they manage after we leave is a puzzle and I like to think they miss us. It's certainly a joyful reunion each time I fill my satchel with pouches of cat food and we descend on the streets that are the special territories of Ginger, Sylvester, Tom Blackie, and all the others. They are stand-ins for our cats at home—our pleasures are busman's holidays—and they are polite, admirable friends in the special way that distinguishes older cats from kittens. Other people fed them too, for we'd see the same faces year after year and nod to them, all members in the great confraternity of cat lovers which crosses any language barrier.

I was especially absorbed in the cats this time because they too have a reputation of cheating the Reaper. If I myself were a cat, instead of just identifying with them as strongly as I do, I'd have said that I was entering on my second life; second of nine. I hoped they could sense and share my exultation.

After cats and flowers and shopping Bill likes fishing, so that's what we did each year on a pier that jutted out into the bay of San Juan. Bill called this fishing ground "the sewer," for the pier is built over what would seem to be a gigantic sewer pipe which discharges its contents at the end. The only others who fished there beside Bill, the "loco Yanqui," were children from "La Perla," the pearl of poverty, one of the poor areas of San Juan. They were bent-pin fishermen and seemed to have every intention of eating their catches but Bill, after frightening Stephanie with promises of bringing home his fish for dinner, would invariably fillet his catch and deliver it to the street cats. Bill fished for pleasure "at the sewer" and he fished in earnest for pompano on the lovely, deserted country beaches to which Dick took us on weekends. I've always loved the tremendous variety of Puerto Rico: a village where bushes are festooned with empty plastic Clorox bottles in a local form of voodoo protection exists just a few miles from a sophisticated tourist paradise with strolling singers and bar stools in the beach huts. It was like living in two different times, two opposite worlds, and we enjoyed ourselves in both; every day, every moment, right up to the end of our stay.

It was Valentine's Day when we returned to a New York hubcap-deep in snow, hopelessly snarled with traffic. No sooner had we checked our city apartment than we started for the country. The main roads had just been cleared but the side roads in Suffolk County were still buried and we crawled along right behind the snowplow. I could barely wait to see our contingent of cats. They all came prancing to greet us, but then I realized that one was missing. Roofles, an orange tabby cat, is our official major-domo: first in the driveway when the car arrives and the very last to see us leave for the city again. Roofles always knew when we were coming, and was out in rain or snow to greet us—but not today. I called him with no result. I turned to Bill. "I don't understand where Roofles can be!" He said, "In the greenhouse, in the barn, somewhere. Maybe the snow is too deep for him." I said, "Roofles always comes!" I called again and again, becoming frightened by the silence. "Roofles isn't here. Where is he?" I began to run, floundering in the snow, out through the garden, all around our property, and near one of the barns I stumbled over a stiff mound in the snow. A protruding tuft of orange fur sent me scrabbling and digging with both hands until I uncovered Roofles: covered with frozen blood, torn, mangled, obviously killed by a dog.

But Roofles was a fighter. Roofles had successfully frightened off most of the dogs in our neighborhood. Roofles was a jealous guardian of our grounds. This wasn't possible! I crouched over the body, remembering the loving, affectionate cat, remembering that we had tried to keep him inside the house with a few of the others while we were gone but had been forced to reassign him to the outside because of his violent disagreements with the inside contingent. If only we'd been able to keep Roofles inside. If only we'd been here a day sooner! A senseless guilt for Roofles's fate was on me, and when Bill raised me to my feet again, I was weeping inconsolably. A pet was lost, a friend was lost, and I was confronted with death again in the midst of my celebration of rebirth.

I cried for Roofles's death. And I cried again many times that afternoon and evening, the tears sluicing down, dimming my eyes. It was hysteria, but also catharsis, a dissolving of months of tension when I had not allowed myself to cry and it left me limp and finally sleepy. I remember Bill pulling the blanket around me.

Around midnight I awoke and decided that I was hungry. I put on a robe and went into the kitchen, but when I switched on a light the room seemed dimmer than usual; another snowstorm "brownout." I turned around—and bumped into a kitchen chair. I opened the refrigerator, took out a carton of orange juice, poured some into a glass, and unaccountably poured too much, flooding the tabletop. I reached for the cleanup sponge on the sink—and missed it. My hand closed on air. I tried again—the sponge was on the left of the faucet—and then I realized that I wasn't seeing anything on my left side—nothing at all. Slowly, I covered my right eye with my hand and there was total darkness. In a flash of terror and disbelief I knew that I could see nothing on the left. I was totally blind in my left eye.

The crying had done it. Freshets of tears had ruptured my eye or detached the retina; even spasms of sneezing could detach a retina. That must be it; but the retina could be fixed, could be surgically reattached, it must be so! Shivering in the warm room, I remembered the other time I'd been carried away on tides of grief. It had happened on another weekend, the weekend that Blynken had been killed, the weekend I'd suffered the burning and squeezing sensations around my heart that were the very first warning of the tumor in my lung. And this was—what? Another warning? Inch by cold inch, fear took me over. It couldn't be related to cancer because the doctors had just declared me cancer-free. All those tests, all those assurances—was it possible they were wrong? Someone had called cancer a mirrored chamber of horrors in which you lived in fear of seeing new terrors unfolding. And this tonight was that horror, wondering whether a detached retina was in fact a detached retina or a metastasis of cancer reaching my brain! Stiffly, carefully, I turned my head, letting the right eye take in all the details of the room. I could see everything that was there, nothing was any worse than it had been a moment ago. The right eye was holding, I was not going completely blind, so it couldn't be a metastasis, could it? No! It was the retina, only the retina. I made myself move though my legs were unwilling, and I started back to the bedroom to awaken Bill. Halfway there, I realized that I wasn't going to waken him now. I had no noble self-sacrificing reason, just a desire not to answer any questions for a while, just a desperate desire for calm. I must be quiet. If I could fall asleep, it might—no, of course it wouldn't—go away in the morning. But in quiet, I could rearm myself with the hard rule that had taken me this far successfully. I began to whisper it: "Don't waste worry. Don't worry until you have all the facts. Learn everything you can and then take action." There was more to this mantra I'd so often repeated, but tonight I could not bring myself to add the rest: "Do not blindly fear." Somehow I reached the bedroom and lay down. In the darkness right eye and left eye were equal. I lay there rigid with fear for a bedmate, but in spite of it, I must have slept a little, for I remember some terrible dreams.

At six, as always, Bill awoke. I heard him washing, heard the buzz of the electric razor and heard him come out of the bathroom, ready to start his day.

"Bill?"

He stopped. He'd heard something in my voice.

"Love, something has happened because of my terrible crying about Roofles. I've damaged my eye. I can't see."

"My God." He was staring into my face. "Which eye?"

"The left."

"I'm calling Doctor Stock right now." He glanced at the clock: six-fifteen. "Doctor Stock has a twenty-four-hour service!" . . . and he was placing the call.

The service answered and said that Doctor Stock was on a skiing vacation and couldn't be reached. Did I want to speak to the doctor who was covering his cases?

I didn't, because the man was a stranger. I wanted someone who knew me, knew my history.

"Let's call Dr. Jaretzki."

We did. He was on vacation, skiing, too.

Bill said, "We have to do something right now. We have to see someone in Southampton." And then he was looking up the number of the doctor we'd always gone to for the minor ailments of the country: colds, sprains, glass cuts, flu. Dr. Merle was on the line immediately.

Our dear kind friend wasted no time on useless questions. He gave us the name of an ophthalmologist in Riverhead who had a fully equipped office in his own home as well as an office in New York. He called that doctor for us. I left the house wearing dark glasses to protect my right eye. The cold was biting but the snowplows had worked late and cleared the roads, so we reached the ophthalmologist's quickly.

He examined my eye, made a series of tests and in a half-hour told me unequivocally that, yes, the retina in my left eye was detached but, yes also, a growth was present there, pressing on my eye. And in view of my malignant lung tumor, he was almost positive that the eye tumor was malignant. But I would have to take a test called an ultrasonogram for the final proof.

We were absolutely silent. Then Bill asked, because I couldn't, "Is the growth operable? Will she see again? Can the retina be reattached?"

"That would be too dangerous until after the tumor is taken care of."

I heard Bill agreeing to the ultrasonogram but declining the doctor's offer to continue beyond that because his New York hospital affiliation was Manhattan Eye and Ear and I preferred to go back to the doctors already familiar with my case, the team at Columbia Presbyterian. The ultrasonogram, I found, was a simple procedure involving the pattern of sonic response through a water-filled, cuplike apparatus fitted over my left eye. The results agreed with the doctor's initial diagnosis: malignancy.

We had celebrated too soon. Puerto Rico was light-years away, our happiness there impossible to imagine, the victory we believed in not mine, but cancer's. And it was so much worse because I thought the struggle was over. I felt betrayed by the tests, by the finest diagnostic instruments, by the doctors' conclusions, all proving nothing but the resurgent power of cancer! Too soon, too soon, I had left my armored shell, let down my guard, relaxed in the sun of rebirth. Now it began again; now I was weary to the bone, discouraged beyond speech.

Back at our house Bill and I could not even speak to each other. We were more dejected, sunk lower than we had been in June, 1974, when we had first learned that I had cancer. This, after we had tried every standard treatment; this, after I had worked so hard, held myself together with such concentration of effort. We'd fought to win and thought we'd won, but I was back among the doomed. Defeated, defeated, nothing now but to go through the motions, repeat it all until the inevitable end. Bill and I both broke a rule we had stringently followed. We cried together that weekend.

Finally Monday came. Finally we were back in the city and on the phone with the chemotherapist, who luckily was in town.

"Absolutely not!" said the chemotherapist. "It can't be malignant. I'll stake my professional reputation on it." He kept on insisting, not only about my course of chemotherapy but also the fact that Dr. Stock had checked me so recently and the tumor would certainly have been detected.

It was a meaningless torrent of words. "I am blind in one eye and the tumor is there," I said. Nothing else meant anything.

It was arranged that I should see a Columbia Presbyterian ophthalmologist. He would schedule another ultrasonogram test, this time in the office of Dr. Coleman Jackson, the inventor of the ultrasonogram. When the ophthalmologist, Dr. L'Esperance, saw me the results were the same, his conclusion identical with that of the Riverhead doctor. A fluke growth was there. A malignancy with a hundred-to-one chance against it. And the ultrasonogram, even when done by a member of Columbia Presbyterian's own club, gave the same diagnosis of malignancy. I had known it would. Only the doctors had to be convinced.

While they were expressing their incredulity, I had made a private decision. If this was what could happen so soon after achieving remission, there was no sense in going the whole tortuous route again. The cancer would only turn up somewhere else in my body and I'd be operated on, take the radiotherapy and the chemotherapy again, suffer all the indignities and the agonies, again, and again, until I was "cured" to bits with each successive cancerous piece of me removed. I'd be like the cancer patients who lingered in hospitals, were let out for a few weeks or months at home, then admitted again for more operations, more postoperative treatments, the fourth, the fifth, sixth, seventh time until their bodies could take no more and they died. But I would not go that way! After Dr. L'Esperance confirmed the diagnosis of malignancy, I told him that I had finished fighting cancer. I did not want to be mutilated bit by bit in the name of cure. I was still alive, still whole, still feeling inexplicably well and I wanted to go on living as fully as I could. Anything that could be done outside the cycle of cut and treat, burn and poison I would accept, but otherwise I would let nature take its course with me. Let nature help me if it could, for I would go on seeking natural remedies, but I was through with the surgical and chemical excesses of the standard treatment. I had lost faith and lost some of my will to fight.

It was a private decision that I did not discuss, even with Bill. He had sacrificed, fought and anguished with me, and even though we had lost, I knew that he could not stop trying, would never accept my attitude. Even now he was steeling himself for the next round.

# CHAPTER XI

# Grand Rounds

My first few days of partial blindness were an exercise in futility. The eye records and sends information to the brain which the brain reinterprets as vision, but both the right and left lenses must focus on an object to perceive depth. Perspective eluded me. I would confidently send out my hand toward the handle of a cup apparently right on target, only to find that my hand was inches away from where I had expected it to be. Slowly I'd "correct," trying to estimate the distance I'd miscalculated. Then, when I sent the hand out to do its job again, I'd mentally allow for the discrepancy, even if it didn't seem right to my eye. Slowly, I trained myself to compensate for the loss of perspective. Slowly, after practice with coffee cups and juice glasses, practice in the sunlight and under the dim lights I would encounter in restaurants, I learned to make the formerly automatic adjustment through careful, but not obvious, concentration.

I didn't intend to allow my loss of sight in one eye to disable me. The problem of sitting with others involved positioning myself without having to swivel my head constantly. There was no seeing my companion to the left; I saw nothing to the left

except the peripheral bit permitted by my right eye. I had to turn
my head completely around to look left or behind, so seating
became very important to me. As long as people were all in
front of me or to my right I could see them perfectly normally,
and I appeared perfectly normal, for my blind left eye looked
and moved just like the right.

More than agility was needed for walking on the street.
Without depth perception one cannot judge the height of a curb
and it's difficult to gauge how close a moving car may be. I
became a rule-book pedestrian, never leading but always following the others on the perilous change of lights.

As I'd imagined, Bill had refused to accept my decision not to
go through standard treatments again. He hadn't refused as
much as he hadn't even listened to me! But I was not operated
on, I did not take chemotherapy, and the doctors came up with a
light schedule of radiotherapy given every day for three weeks,
a "reasonable" 1,000 rads, as they put it. Cancer therapy is
extremely casual in its use of big numbers. The seriousness of
the situation becomes apparent in the outcry raised about exposing women to the one or one and a half rads needed in mammog-
raphy, the X-ray test to detect breast cancer. But I committed
myself to this "reasonable" radiotherapy again; partly because
Bill almost shouted at me, "We'll do what we have to do and
now it's eye radiation!" and partly because the doctors held out
the very good possibility of regaining my sight afterward. When
the tumor had been killed, then I could consider an operation to
reattach my retina.

And that was not the only carrot held out to me. A week after
the discovery of the tumor in my eye, Dr. Stock came back from
his skiing vacation—a vacation he had shared with Dr. Jaretzki,
I discovered—and was honestly nonplussed to find me where I
was. He consulted immediately with Dr. L'Esperance, the
latest doctor added to my train. Dr. Stock could not seem to get
over the indisputable fact that a month ago he had examined me

and a month ago he had seen nothing. "I am not an ophthal-mologist, of course," he finally remarked. I looked at him, wondering if he meant that I should have parceled myself out to specialists and asked an ophthalmologist to do that part of the examination. Certainly it had never occurred to me that safety lay in overlapping doctors! Dr. Stock approved the course of "light" radiation I was taking, but he seemed to be looking for something else I could do, some other way of explaining the incredible existence of my incredible tumor.

"There is a forum held at the Vanderbilt Institute that I think you should visit," he told me. "It's called the Grand Rounds. We'll arrange for you to go there."

The Vanderbilt Institute, I knew, was the Eye and Ear division associated with Columbia Presbyterian and I had an im-mediate picture of a symposium, a special gathering of eye doctors who would examine patients referred to them by other doctors. Out of such a large group of specialists, there might very well be a useful opinion that could be applied to my present condition or to the surgery I'd need later to reattach my retina. The Grand Rounds, by all means! At four in the afternoon of the following Thursday, Bill and I would be at the Vanderbilt Institute, waiting for the Grand Rounds to begin.

We were there half an hour early and surprised not to find some notice about this special event. The elevator operator seemed baffled: "You mean the clinic?" "The Grand Rounds," we insisted. Well, he said, he didn't know but he took us to the floor we wanted and suggested that we wait. We did wait, alone, in a dingy space scarcely wider than a cor-ridor—I think it *was* a corridor—and eventually we began to explore some deserted conference rooms. Layers of New York soot proved that nothing had been cleaned in weeks. "We must be on the wrong floor," Bill said. And actually we tried asking questions of people on several other floors but the vagueness of their responses to "Grand Rounds" brought us back to our original corridor. A nurse was passing by. We hurried after her, asking where the conference of ophthalmologists would be held. "Just wait right here, they'll be along," she said, and left us. We brushed off the seats of two chairs with handkerchiefs and sat down. Then, gradually, people began to wander off the elevator. First there was an old man whose stumbling feet needed guidance from the young boy with him; then a frail old lady with a bandaged eye; several pale, desiccated wearers of dark glasses; someone partially blind with a cane, someone else with a turban of bandages—yes, these were obviously patients, but where were the doctors? I saw no one resembling a doctor but noticed a frizzy-haired young man in sweater and jeans taking people's names. Close up, he had an impressive crop of pimples. "Are you part of the Grand Rounds?" I asked. "Yes, yes," he answered. "This is the clinic. Are you here for the clinic?" he asked quizzically.

I looked around. A few other young men had materialized. One or two seemed coordinated enough to be doctors in practice but the rest ambled about like scraggly hippie visitors; disheveled—no—they were dirty! And there wasn't a cleanup sink in sight.

"Bill?" I quavered.

"It's the clinic," said my husband. "And it's the Grand Rounds, too."

True, fine ophthalmologists from Columbia Presbyterian might come to devote part of their time here, certainly medical students came to "observe" and interns to practice, but I had no intention of submitting to their apparently casual probings. One of the grimier young men was working his way down the line of patients toward us. "He'd better not try to touch my face," I said. "I just saw him remove the dressing from that man's eye and it was running with some kind of matter. He hasn't even washed his hands!"

I don't know if the absolute lack of hygiene bothered anyone else as much as it did me, but I had only one good eye to guard from contamination. I jumped up. As we hurried away I thought that at least the patients with cataracts and bandaged eyes couldn't see the condition of the clinic—or of their doctors—clearly enough to worry.

For some stubborn reason of my own I decided to say nothing to Dr. Stock about this colossal flop. He mentioned the matter a few weeks later, after my eye radiotherapy had ended. "Well, did you ever get to the Grand Rounds?"

"Grand Rounds?" I scoffed. "They were more like the Dirty Dozen." And I gave him the complete rundown.

He roared with laughter. "Now you're getting to see some of the strange aspects of medicine today. But in spite of the way things looked, there was a lot of talent there."

"If they were so dedicated to medicine, why didn't they have more respect for their patients? Do you pick a pimple and then lay your hands on someone's eyes? Doctor Stock, you're on the Admitting Board of the Columbia Medical School. Why don't you take a close look at what you're letting in these days? Or go down to the Grand Rounds. See for yourself."

He smiled and let it drop.

Why had he even suggested it? I had an uncharitable explanation for my good doctor's deviousness: either he wanted to divert my mind with a new hope of recovery or he simply wanted the students to get a look at my case. I'd been told often enough that everything about my case was uncommon. My cancer's revealing itself as it had was a fluke, my general health and resistance to X-ray side effects was a fluke, and what had happened to my eye after all the previous treatment was both a fluke and an impossibility. It's likely that I rated high as an educational exhibit for the learners. But I realized that Dr. Stock's unimpeachable integrity was one reason why he was the doctor I most trusted and he would never play such games.

I knew that my momentary suspicion of Dr. Stock's motive

arose out of a sad recognition that the cancer patient has a peculiar status in medicine. He loses his personal rights because he is a mine of involuntary information. What he can "take" in the way of treatment holds clues for a future cancer cure and what he may feel while "taking it" is most casually handled— after all, he has cancer and no choice but to endure. A cancer patient is not dead, but he may be dying, and he's certainly removed at least one step from the rest of humanity. A glass wall of fatal statistics separates him from the world; communication between the two tends to be muffled and poor. I had this depersonification demonstrated to me again during the radiotherapy treatments for my eye.

This time I had no real discomfort. The radiotherapist reiterated that the 1,000 rads I was getting in my left temple was a light dose but sufficien to kill the tumor, and my hope that my sight would eventually be restored was not at all unreasonable. She put it much more strongly than that: she felt I had real, legitimate hope. I was just beginning to feel confident and cared for again when I arrived one day to take my treatment and found that the monster machine was "on the blink" like any toaster. Experts from California had flown in to repair it and I waited two or three days until the hospital called and said I could resume my treatment. I was halfway through the session on the slab when the technician turned off the machine, darted out of her safety booth and began to check switches and make computations. "Oh hell," I heard her mutter, "it's out again."

"What do you mean?" I demanded. "Did something happen while I was on the machine?"

She nodded. "Didn't you hear that noise?"

I had heard something slightly different from the program of sounds the machine emitted during its operation but the deviation—no warning "ping," no rasp of gears—had not really registered on my nontechnical mind. But what the technician said next really did alarm me. One of the machine's automatic systems had not been repaired. The California experts were returning next week to finish the job and for now the hospital technicians were making manual corrections for the machine's inaccuracies . . . yet the hospital had called me back to resume my treatment! I almost shouted at her: "Would you have gone on the machine knowing there was an automatic malfunction that was being corrected by hand?"

She said she would not.

"Then why do you presume that I would?"

Of course she did not answer that; of course she did not say what I myself was thinking: Because you have cancer you have no choice. But no one had troubled to tell me in advance and I found out only by asking further that it had happened not once but three times. Three times while I was taking treatment, while it was sending rays into my brain, the monster had malfunctioned. I was simply told that "these things happen." I was told that the malfunction had nothing to do with the dosage, that I was in no danger, that "they" knew how to cope with it. It was all casually passed over but I remember every word. I had fought like a madwoman for over six months to save my life, to avoid taking extra risks! Now, I felt anger, sorrow, futility, and resentment, but could they understand the strength of my feelings on the other side of that glass wall?

There was nothing to do after the radiotherapy but wait the appropriate length of time until we could see if the tumor had been killed and then face the problem of an operation to restore my sight. I had improved my skills as a one-eyed woman. I was reading books and magazines almost as quickly as I had before, I was pouring without spilling, and I had mastered the seating ballet in restaurants and other people's homes. Nothing pleased me more than to have the person I had been lunching with for half an hour stare earnestly at me and finally ask, "But which eye is it, Joie?" I always told the truth, and always reassured myself afterward by looking in the mirror. Yes, the eye moved normally with the other, sighted, one; the eyebrows and eyelashes were still intact, having survived the second round of radiotherapy. But even with my normal outward appearance I had a new sense of growing nervousness.

I didn't want anything to happen to my precious right eye. I gave up driving. It had been a bravura performance, I suppose, good only till the next examination for renewal of my license. I'd been proud of the way I'd managed, keeping to the slower right lane on the highways, checking my side mirror constantly, parking carefully on the right. But now it was making both Bill and me uneasy. Suppose a piece of dust flew in, suppose a sudden stop sent my head against the windshield—no, it was easier to stop entirely. Bill fretted about the odd accident—the fragment of rock, the snapping twig—and told me well in advance that he would not allow me to prune the roses next summer. Privately, I worried about my occasional headaches on the right side. Was it just inevitable eyestrain from using one eye to compensate for two or was it, could it be metastasis, the same thing again?

My doctors assured me that tumors did not duplicate themselves in that way. There was no basis for belief in a "sympathetic occurrence." It would not happen again.

But the doctors had assured me of so many things. I learned some months later, when I checked into the Janker Clinic in Germany, that the "legitimate hope" for the restoration of sight in my left eye had vanished on the monster X-ray machine. Not because of its tendency to malfunction, but because of the strength of the radiation I had been given. To the German doctors, the metastasis to the eye was not such a fluke; they observed it as a frequent occurrence in lung cancers like mine. And they were able to restore sight to the affected eye most of the time, treating it with chemotherapy and the most minute amounts of radiation. I had been exposed to far more radiation than they ever used. Did I say that I'd been given 1,000 rads? So

I'd been told, many times. But when I was able to pry loose my American hospital records for the German doctors' use, I found that I had not been told the truth and that someone else had made a decision about my life without informing me. My hospital records proved that I had been given not 1,000 rads, but 3,000. This was an amount guaranteed to kill the tumor—it did kill the tumor—and also it completely burned out my eye. No operation could help. I would never see with my left eye again.

If someone had presented me with the choice of taking 3,000 rads because it was the only sure way to kill the tumor or taking less than 1,000 rads, which might well enable me to see again but also might not finish off the tumor conclusively, then I don't know what I would have answered. I might have avoided the choice entirely and said that I'd seek an alternative mode of treatment somewhere in the world. But I was never asked, never informed that the dilemma existed, never given the chance to say, "No, I'll go elsewhere!" It was incredible ignorance or arrogance on the part of the doctors who prescribed and administered the treatment. I had apparently become a laboratory animal to them. I was more aware of the loss of my rights than ever before. For a moment I considered suing "them," but only for a moment. I had the most to lose in such a suit; I needed to focus my whole concentration on survival, to pour my positive energy into the search for a cure. It was over and my eye was dead. But I would not be "done unto" any longer. I would choose my own course. No one would ever make decisions for me again.

# CHAPTER XII

# Enzymes and Embryos

Wobe Mugos is not an incantation, it is a biochemical formula recommended by a science-writer friend when he heard of my case. The enzyme-based drug had been developed by Dr. Max Wolf, who was, at ninety-five, semi-retired from practice, but my friend was sure that he could easily be persuaded to help.

Dr. Wolf was still very active in cancer research. He had come to this interest through the study of degenerative diseases in his original specialty of geriatrics. From the rejuvenation of the aging celebrities who had been his original patients, he had moved toward the goal of retarding undesirable changes in human cells, and now spent six months of every year in Germany working with cancer patients, further developing the enzyme therapy that he claimed had an immunological force against cancer.

I called Dr. Wolf's Florida home in late March of 1975. A strong, sympathetic voice answered the phone. Of course he would see me. I would not have to come to Florida, he would be returning to White Plains, just outside New York, in about a week. I could make an appointment now.

I tried to think of a considerate hour for a man of his age. "Is ten o'clock too early, Doctor?"

I heard him laughing. "I see patients at five A.M. when it is necessary. Please don't worry about me. What will be convenient for you?"

I was excited, and used the intervening week to read about enzyme therapy. The concept of enzyme healing is ancient: the Indian medicine men who put papaya leaves and flowers on patients' wounds were making use of the healing enzymes in papaya; Chinese medicinal "broths" contained plants whose enzymes speeded healing in interior infections. And today's medicine knows the nature of enzyme chemistry, though not all its diverse functions and possibilities. Enzymes are natural catalytic agents, produced by living cells, which accelerate and change body processes. They are responsible for the day-to-day state of digestion, the peculiarities of metabolism, the aging of cells and the degenerative changes in organs. Enzymes regulate changes, and it seemed to me a natural, logical step to make enzymes work in cancer therapy to retard undesirable changes in the cells. Work in enzyme biochemistry apparently began in earnest around the turn of the twentieth century with a man named J. Beard. Other researchers followed, among them the man I was to meet, Dr. Max Wolf.

Bill drove me to Dr. Wolf's house in White Plains the following week. He decided to wait in the car. After all, the enzyme formula Dr. Wolf dispensed to his patients was still illegal in this country, though in standard use in Europe, and perhaps he might be reluctant to give it in the presence of two perfect strangers. We had learned caution in Chinatown!

I had been expecting a stern Teuton and I found Santa Claus. The thick, springy crepe soles of his beige suede shoes didn't raise him to my eye level. He had very bright blue eyes, very rosy cheeks, firm skin and almost no wrinkles and the engaging remains of an Austrian accent. I couldn't avoid thinking of words like "elf," "sprite" and "St. Nicholas."

I followed the doctor through a room hung with magnificent sixteenth-century art and into a study. He said, "Tell me about the treatments you are getting now, please," as he took notes in the tiniest imaginable scrawl. I detailed my story. He said that the radiation and chemotherapy I'd taken did not "show," the effects had probably been beneficial, and that I seemed to be free of the usual disturbances that went with the treatments. I waited for him to tell me I looked "well and healthy," as so many people did, but Doctor Wolf knew better. He had dealt with hundreds of cancer patients and appreciated the complete unpredictability of the disease. When he had finished his notations he began to tell me about Wobe Mugos and the enthusiasm that gradually crept into his voice told me how deeply he believed in the possibilities of his therapy.

Wobe Mugos, Dr. Wolf said, is a protease mixture, a mixture of enzymes that break down into complex chemical substances and can inhibit the development of inflammation. This is the basis of its healing action. Proteases or, as Dr. Wolf consistently called them, proteolytic enzymes, do not affect healthy living cells, but do have an as yet uncharted effect on viruses. Wobe Mugos consisted of enzymes extracted from plant and animal components: beef pancreas, calf thymus, lens esculenta, pisum sativum, papyotin and mannit from figs, papaya and other plant life. After years of research, this was the best combination Dr. Wolf had found in treatment of degenerative diseases.

"Can you give me an example of how Wobe Mugos might apply to cancer?"

Dr. Wolf cited the condition of the pancreas in cancer patients. "Enzymes direct, accelerate, modify or retard all body functions. Thus, absence or insufficiency of one or several enzymes would naturally lead to disturbance or dysfunction in the body. The pancreas is of paramount importance to digestion and metabolism and yet, every cancer patient invariably has some degree of pancreatic deficiency. The function of Wobe Mugos therapy would be to substitute the missing enzymatic action and compensate for the pancreatic deficiency.''

''You're trying to keep the organs of the body in a working balance,'' I said.

He nodded. ''Yes, I view cancer as a disease that involves the whole body. Neither of the classic approaches, surgery or radioactive therapy, the knife or the rays, can produce a complete recovery from cancer in most cases, because the thing they attack, the tumor itself, is only a symptom of the disease. Cancer must be treated as a disease of the total body. The body must help to heal itself.''

''How, Doctor?''

With references to a chart and textbook illustrations, Dr. Wolf began to explain how the cancer cell disguises itself to elude the normal defenses of the body. Each cancer cell is covered with a sticky material which disguises its nature as an outsider and enables it to adhere to a surface and grow without interruption until it becomes a tumor. But enzyme therapy, Dr. Wolf told me, can strip the protective sticky covering from the cancer cell and thus enable the body's defensive leucocytes to invade and destroy it. Further, since already formed tumors ''shed'' cancer cells which circulate through the bloodstream and adhere to host cells elsewhere to form new cancerous colonies of metastases, the raising of the levels of proteolytic enzymes in the blood should prevent the formation of these metastases by making it impossible for the cancer cells to attach themselves anywhere.

My comprehension of the doctor's theory of therapy was limited, but I understood enough to make me tremble with hope as I received my first injection of Wobe Mugos. And I was relieved to learn that it was available in capsule form; I could take it at home.

Dr. Wolf told me that there were various methods of administering Wobe Mugos, but my home supply was a retention enema tablet or rectal clysma. My Wobe Mugos kit was a syringe with a small plastic tube, a Lucite box with fifty capsules and an instruction leaflet in German. (The Wobe Mugos was prepared in Germany by a firm in which Dr. Wolf had a partnership, a fact that originally gave me pause in my evaluation of the treatment.)

My instructions for home treatments were as follows: every twelve hours, place three capsules in the tube, add about 10 ccs. of warm water, shake the mixture vigorously until it dissolved completely, then draw it into the syringe. Then lie on the left side, insert the syringe into the rectum, depress the plunger and rest in position for twenty minutes. This procedure had to be repeated twice a day, every day, for the next thirty days, and after that, on alternate days.

The fifty-capsule package of Wobe Mugos, approximately enough for one week during the first month of treatment, enough for two weeks thereafter, cost seventy-five dollars. Expensive, certainly, but still I thought I'd better stockpile a supply since Doctor Wolf might return to Florida or go to Europe. He assured me that he'd have whatever I needed sent to me from Germany if necessary. And he gave me cautionary instructions to keep the capsules away from moisture: it caused deterioration. I decided to keep them in my bedside drawer and tape the seams of the Lucite box with adhesive to insure a dry environment inside.

"About your diet while you are taking Wobe Mugos" . . . Dr. Wolf began to tick off the prohibited foods on the fingers of his small hand. "No alcohol. No animal fats. No fermentative foods such as bread, cheese or wine. Absolutely no white sugar." I said, "Oh, the Freund Cancerphobe diet. I know it, I've been on it."

"Good, then you are set."

"When do I see you again, Doctor?"

"The same time next week. Please bring in your X-rays, both before and after the radiation treatments. And I would like to see a pathology report."

I rose to go and he accompanied me to the door. "If you follow this enzyme therapy, I believe that we will be able to stop metastases and bring about some improvement in the pancreas deficiency." Casually, he added, "There is also a bonus, Mrs. McGrail. You will notice a wonderful feeling of well-being in a few days. Perhaps even euphoria."

I froze in place. Euphoria to me meant a prescription from a Dr. Feelgood, a prescription with an addictive quotient that brings "highs" and "lows" to the patient, making him slavishly dependent on the dosage.

"Dr. Wolf . . ." I began.

He looked at my suspicious face.

"Is there anything in Wobe Mugos that is addictive?" I asked.

"But I have told you what is in it."

"Is there anything you didn't tell me?"

He laughed. "No, no, please do not worry, there is nothing addictive or dangerous. Remember, we use Wobe Mugos in Europe not only for cancer, but for a whole range of other conditions, for degeneration of tissue, for circulation problems . . . no, it is all natural and wholesome. You can take it without my supervision for a long time without any problem at all."

"Then what about the euphoria?"

"That comes because the poisons are flushed from the tumor site and taken out of your body. Of course you would feel better."

We shook hands briskly, European-style, and I went back to the car.

Well?'' Bill demanded. "Is he legitimate?''

"I don't know, but he believes in his enzyme therapy completely, I am sure of that. I believe that Wobe Mugos is worth trying. It may truly help me, and if it doesn't, it certainly can't hurt.''

Bill worried and fretted all the way back to the city as I repeated what Doctor Wolf had told me. He was most impressed by the fact that the Wobe Mugos enzymes did not cause any changes in healthy tissue and could, if necessary, be taken with antibiotics. It seemed to prove their harmlessness. By the time we pulled into our garage, I had won Bill over to my "Might help. Can't hurt" point of view.

I began the treatment. After a few days there was what I can only describe as a "cleaner" feeling, more energy, a sense of clearer focus. Each day I felt better. I began to bloom, expand, relax, let my natural optimism out of its cautionary box. Other people could see a difference in me, and then I began to feel a surge in vitality, a quickening that was almost like old times. Was this my answer? I felt so well that first week that Dr. Wolf's reaction to my X-rays at our second appointment was doubly disappointing, doubly chilling.

He studied them somberly. "There is a wonderful clinic in Bonn," he said at last. "They use a very potent chemotherapy that is not available in the United States. I think you should go there and take it.''

"Why? I am in remission," I protested. "I've just had a blood test. I've had recent X-rays. I know I am in remission.''

Gently, very gently, he answered me. "Remission can last six months, six years, or six weeks. It means that you have reached a plateau, but . . .'' The word trailed off warningly.

"I thought I was finished with hospitals!''

Doctor Wolf looked away from me. Knowing what he knew

about cancer, he could surmise what lay in store for me and for almost all cancer patients. My defiance was futile. But he only said:

"For the future, it is necessary to safeguard against any possible activity of that large tumor in your lung. And there have been metastases, too."

"I'm aware of that, Doctor."

"Mrs. McGrail, the clinic in Bonn, the Janker Klinik, is, in my opinion, the best in the world. If you were my mother or my sister or my wife"—he paused to blink away the very real tears that glistened in his eyes—"I would beg you to go!"

He said no more and it would have done little good; I wasn't really listening. I didn't want to hear about the end of a remission, I was in it, I had made it, and in my mind I was determined to give Wobe Mugos a chance to work. If it worked, I might be free of hospitals forever.

After three weeks of the Wobe Mugos treatments, I had trouble remembering to rest in the afternoon. On April 21, 1975, Bill and I celebrated my fifty-third birthday with the zest of youngsters. We went out on the town, I collected compliments, we were irrepressible as he toasted me in champagne and I replied in apple juice. Wonderful Wobe Mugos! A clinic in Bonn could have been on Mars.

On April 22, in Dr. Wolf's office for a routine checkup, I asked him if there was anything I could do to insure the continuity of the exuberant well-being.

"Have you ever heard of Dr. Hans Neihans?"

"You mean the Neihans cellular therapy in Switzerland?"

I could hardly believe it. It was my private wish since I was an editor at *Harper's Bazaar* and we ran the first articles on the cellular therapy that regenerated and rejuveniated Churchill, Adenauer, Pope Pius XI, and other very rich or very important people. I had promised to treat myself to Dr. Neihans's magic before I was sixty. And although it might be happening under unexpectedly grim circumstances, the old excitement and curiosity surfaced. I looked at Dr. Wolf's firm ninety-five-year-old cheeks and wondered if he was a Neihans graduate too.

"Were you close friends?"

"Oh yes. In fact, I gave him the injections, and at his clinic they were administered without local anesthetic. Very painful. You hoped for a friendly hand."

"What could the Neihans cellular therapy do for me medically?"

"It would help to rebuild debilitated organs and do so very specifically. It is amazing—the embryonic material has a sort of "homing instinct"; lung cells go straight to the lungs, heart cells to the heart. Science cannot yet explain why."

"When can I take the treatment?"

"Wait, wait. First you take the Abderhalden tests. They will indicate, through the urine, which of your organs needs help."

I suddenly remembered that the Neihans treatments cost the earth. Ten thousand dollars was the price in the early days! I asked if conditions had changed.

"Definitely. Live embryos were put into immediate use then—removed from pregnant sheep while the patient waited to receive them on the operating table. It was complicated, there was a great problem with infection and sometimes diseases were passed along from the animal to the patient. But since then a way had been found to immediately dry-freeze the embryo material and the cost has greatly decreased."

Another factor concerned me. "Doctor, if I take the Neihans cellular therapy, how long would I have to stay in Switzerland?"

"Not a minute." He enjoyed my confusion. "I'm going to give you the cell injections right here."

I broke out in a verbal rash of questions. Did he mean in his office? Was he sure he would have the different kinds of cells needed for whatever organs of mine the test showed needed reinforcement? How about reaction with the Wobe Mugos? Could I go home immediately? How long would I have to stay in bed?

"Wait, wait!" Up went his hand in protest, cutting off my questions. "I promise to tell you everything. You will get the cell injections here and rest at home for the balance of the day. Take no baths for three days. Absolutely no alcohol for at least one week. And yes, I have all the cell material we will need, enough to cover every possible result of the Abderhalden test. There will be no problem!"

Dr. Wolf explained that the Abderhalden Reactions (Tests for Specific Organ-Antienzymes) provided an analysis of the condition of every organ and gland in the human body through the analysis of the urine. Although the urinanalysis method of gauging health and detecting disease is a standard medical procedure, Professor E. Abderhalden, a biologist of the University of Halle, Switzerland, developed a method of determining the extent of damage to each affected part. The results of the Abderhalden tests indicate the condition of organs and glands on a scale ranging from normal to slightly abnormal, moderately abnormal, distinctly abnormal and markedly abnormal.

My report of April, 1975, showed my pancreas, lungs, eye, pericardium, lymph glands and hypophysis all distinctly abnormal, my liver and hypothalmus moderately abnormal, and my heart, pleuria, glie cells and arteries slightly abnormal. I received dry sheep embryo pancreas, liver, lung, eye and lymph cells without any pain or side effects. I marveled that the cells would all race to reinforce that organ of mine which corresponded to the same organ in the unborn sheep.

I don't know how—or if—the Neihans cellular therapy benefited me. I do know that my energy and general condition were excellent and that my psychological and mental frames were positive and strong and that it was a very good summer in 1975.

But I couldn't forget Dr. Wolf's grave warning that remission can be a fleeting reprieve. And hadn't I lost an eye to a malignant tumor in the midst of celebrating my *last* remission? I could not let my guard down again. I could not rest here. I must go on in spite of my dread to whatever next terrible step lay ahead.

*CHAPTER XIII*

# Seeking Therapies
# in Other Lands

"But Doctor Wolf has written to Dr. Hoefer about me. My arrival here has all been arranged."

"Please?" The lanky blonde with the flyaway hair obviously didn't understand. We stood there, Bill and I, beside our pile of luggage in the cold, empty vestibule of 12-14 Baumschulallee, Bonn.

"I am expected," I began again. "We have just arrived from New York. I am to be a patient at the Janker Klinik. Dr. Wolf has arranged it with Dr. Hoefer. . . ."

"Herr Doktor Hoefer?" She nodded comprehension. "Herr Doktor Hoefer ist nicht hier."

"You're not expected and the doctor's not here," Bill said grimly.

We'd had our misgivings at the first sight of the rambling yellow frame building. It looked rundown, vaguely seedy and we doubted that the cab driver had, in fact, delivered us to the address written out on the slip of paper we had handed him at the airport. Finally he stumped out of his cab and pointed to a small brass plaque beside the front door: JANKER STRAHLENKLINIK. Impatiently, he began to remove our luggage. Bill tried the bell. The door opened quickly on a blinking, middle-aged man who simply stood there until the taxi driver advanced past him and dumped our luggage on the floor of the vestibule.

"Janker Klinik?" Bill asked.

The man moved aside to let us pass. Behind him was the empty hall and a deserted wooden desk.

"Let's keep the taxi," said Bill. "I think there's been a mistake."

He turned to the driver, whose hand was outstretched for payment.

"How do you say 'Wait for me' in German?"

I couldn't help. The Berlitz book of German phrases was somewhere in our luggage.

Bill began speaking English very loudly and slowly and the taxi driver answered equally loudly and slowly in German so that we would surely understand. Bill opened his wallet and enlisted the driver's very close attention. He paid our fare in Deutschmarks—it was more than thirty dollars for the ride from the airport—and then took out a few more bills. Waving them back and forth for emphasis, he intoned, "Wait for us. Wait in the taxi. Wait till we come."

The driver gestured, unmistakably the motion of the meter running.

"Okay. Yes. Ja," said Bill.

As the driver went outside, we turned to the man, who must have been a combination porter and receptionist.

"Sprechen Sie Englisch?"

"Nein," said the man promptly. "Parlez-vous français?"

Bill looked at me, but any shred of French fled in confusion. Bill finally put together a circuitous paragraph about finding the right person to whom we could speak, the doctor's secretary, perhaps . . . the "secrétaire"?

It was a lucky word. He crossed to the receptionist's desk and pressed a button on the switchboard. "Secrétaire, Sekretärin," he said proudly, filling in the language gap.

Moments later, the blonde with the flyaway hair confronted us.

This was Doctor Hoefer's secretary. But she was not expecting us. And Doctor Hoefer was not here.

"Will the doctor be back soon?" I ventured.

She struggled and found her English. "In a little while he comes."

"Let's wait, Bill," I said. But Bill never likes to wait and I could see that the apparent disorganization around us was making him nervous. "Suppose you stay here until Doctor Hoefer comes and I'll take our luggage to a hotel."

"No, No!" said the blonde suddenly. "No hotel rooms in Bonn. Not one! Big convention today and tomorrow. All room been taken." Our accommodations were to have been made by the clinic.

Bill began to take on an expression that I knew meant we might be barreling back to the airport headed for the next New York flight at any moment.

"Bill, I have my X-rays and all my records. By the time Dr. Hoefer gets here and I've finished showing them to him, I'm sure you'll be back. Why don't you go now? That meter's still running."

I followed the secretary through a labyrinth of corridors and cut-up rooms divided by wooden partitions. She moved at a nervous lope, and since I had recently sprained my right foot, I had trouble keeping up with her. We passed several enormous partitioned-off areas, apparently X-ray departments, for technicians were shuttling in and out with prints in hand. There was haste everywhere; everything seemed to be done on the double; and everything was bare and Spartan: plain wooden cubicles, rooms with curtains instead of doors, steep wooden staircases spiraling up to the other floors. There was a touch of hysteria to the Janker staff's style—''dashing and flapping'' I called it later—and it was a blend of too much work, too few people to do it and the genuine conviction that ''macht schnell'' meant more devotion to duty.

Fortunately, Dr. Hoefer's office was an island of calm. He returned after I had been waiting only a few moments: a tall, courtly man who seemed to fold in half as he bowed over my hand and murmured polite German greetings. His hair was a tight silver helmet, his eyes deeply shadowed by fatigue. Dr. Hoefer was the owner of Janker Klinik and one of the top oncologists in the world. He at least had been expecting me. Of course hotel accommodations for my stay as a Klinik outpatient should have been arranged. Of course! But—he sighed with heavy Prussian gravity—the secretary had so much work to do, there were so many papers on her desk. Mine were probably at the bottom of the pile, I thought. I did not have much confidence in the galloping blonde's abilities and even less in Dr. Hoefer's description of her as ''speaking good English.'' His own English, which he pronounced exactly as if it were German, was hard enough to follow. There was plenty of leeway for misunderstandings. Communication would be a problem here.

Dr. Stock had asked me not to open my X-rays and records until I gave them to Dr. Hoefer and I'd been faithful to my promise. I gave Dr. Hoefer the sealed packet and I watched him in silence as he flipped through the papers and studied the X-rays without comment. He did not look at them long, but rose suddenly and said it was time for me to begin at Janker: X-rays first and chemical tests afterward. As I followed him back through the maze of corridors toward the X-ray department, my right ankle was paining me so sharply that I had to lean heavily on the cane I carried.

On the way to the X-ray department we met Bill, who was full of cheer and accomplishment.

"There are two big conventions in town and the hotels are full, but we have a quiet room with balcony and bath in the best hotel in Bonn."

Bill always manages these little miracles, but I pretended to be very much surprised.

I noticed that the Janker's X-ray department had a wooden door that separated the area of X-ray machines from the bare cubicles where patients waited. But the door hung badly on its frame and there were large open spaces at the bottom. I shuddered at the idea of unnecessary exposure to X-rays; I had an impulse to stuff my clothes into those cracks! But I was the only one who seemed perturbed. Another missing "frill" was the usual hospital smock: both men and women went bare-breasted into X-ray. I looked around and saw that no one, large or small, seemed to feel the least self-consciousness: only I, American and embarrassed, wished that I had not chosen to wear maroon-colored knickers and high patent-leather boots that day. I felt like a topless circus poster, and it was a very long walk across the big room to X-ray when my turn came.

The X-ray procedure was developed in Germany and advanced work continues here. Television X-ray scanning diagnostics were pioneered at Janker Klinik and after the usual X-rays, I was taken to another room and put through a series of very intricate scans by Dr. Hoefer.

As Bill and I sat waiting for the results in Dr. Hoefer's office we agreed that coming to Janker was a good form of insurance for the future. We knew that the tumor in my left lung, and one hoped its attendant nodules, had been burned and blasted into scar tissue, but there would be millions of cancer cells too small to be detected still alive in my body. The potent German chemical therapy for which we had journeyed here would dispose of those cells before they grew. The chemical used was Trophosphamide, not available in the United States because the FDA considered it too dangerous. And it *was* dangerous but so was my inoperable cancer. Trophosphamide had added years to cancer patients' lives and produced remissions so complete that they might almost be called cures, but it had also caused many deaths, especially in the early years of experimentation on consenting terminal patients. Trophosphamide had a propensity of causing hemorraghic cystitis and completely destroying the kidneys. When the kidneys failed to function and the toxic residue of Trophosphamide remained in the body, the patient died. Finally a treatment was devised at Janker Klinik to sharply minimize the likelihood of kidney failures. But another problem still remained in Trophosphamidal therapy. Because of the chemical's overwhelming potency, the patient's white-cell blood count temporarily falls to a level considered lethal by most doctors in most countries. During the critical ten-day period after taking Trophosphamide, the white-cell blood count might fall well below 1,000, all the way down to an impossible 300. Still, patient after patient was now surviving this rigorous cure and Janker Klinik was besieged by desperately anxious people who wanted the therapy.

Hating chemotherapy as I did, I had gone through some fairly involved mental calisthenics to get myself to Bonn. I knew that Trophosphamide was supremely effective, and I assumed that I would not need a massive dose of chemicals and not have to endure any deep radiation because my tumor was already dead. At my core, I knew that I had come because Dr. Max Wolf, whose enzyme therapy had so improved my general condition, had told me that I must. Not once, but many times he had said that the two or three weeks I would spend at the Janker Klinik would be my next necessary step toward recovery.

Dr. Hoefer returned with his colleague and Klinik Direktor, Dr. Wolfgang Scheef. Dr. Scheef, a wiry, energetic man, spoke excellent English. He placed my new X-rays in a viewing box and pointed to an area in my right lung.

"Mrs. McGrail, there is a spot here. You see? I would call it the size of a summer pea."

I jumped up immediately, ignoring the pain in my ankle. "Dr. Scheef, there's a mistake. These can't be my X-rays. My tumor is in the left lung, not the right!"

He shook his head. "We have seen the tumor site in your left lung. It shows no activity and that is marvelous. But this—this is a metastasis to the right lung. We feel sure that we will be able to kill this new tumor in the course of your treatment here."

One month ago, only one month ago, in New York, in October, X-rays of my lungs were taken as part of my regular checkup. And one month ago no spot had been seen in my right lung. Or was that true? I became frantic with sudden suspicions. Why had Dr. Stock made me promise not to look at my records before I presented them to Dr. Hoefer? Why had they been sealed? Had my doctors at Columbia Presbyterian seen the new tumor and made still another "decision for my own good," keeping it secret from me, knowing that I would find out in Germany? Was it possible that the radiologist in New York had concentrated on my left lung with its known tumor and neglected to look at my right? No, impossible. But that very refutation opened the way to something much more sinister: suppose there *was* no tumor in my right lung a month ago. If its growth had accelerated so hideously in only four weeks, then I was doomed unless I took whatever the Janker Klinik had to offer and took it immediately! To kill the tumor there would be higher dosages of the dangerous drug; to kill the tumor there would be deep radiation again burning through my body.

The doctors told me how they would proceed. For the first week I would be an outpatient, coming to the Klinik only for a daily dose of cobalt radiation. ("It's far below the levels you're accustomed to at home," Dr. Scheef told me. "We only toast you gently here.") And then I would enter the Klinik as a regular patient to take the Trophosphamide therapy. But I'd be there not for the two weeks Dr. Wolf had suggested, but for six weeks at least: long enough to emerge from the critical ten-day period, long enough so that my white-cell count would return to normal levels, long enough to take any adjunct therapy necessary, to see whether any new tumor activity could be detected with the finest of diagnostic instruments. Bill would be staying in the hotel only a block and a half away. We looked at each other; the block and a half was a chasm, another world.

The first week we pretended that we were free. The cobalt treatment took only a little of my time each day and produced no complications or side effects. There was lots of time to become depressed by our situation, and to avoid doing so, we decided to explore the mysteries of Bonn. Bonn is probably one of the world's grayest and stodgiest towns, with a chill winter drizzle that slicks the cobblestones of the old streets to a treacherous smoothness. We walked as much as I was able, as carefully as I could, and found the lovely medieval plaza with its outdoor markets and tiny, enticing shops. We bought vegetables, greenhouse flowers and pretty things to cheer ourselves. And then we found a particularly German treat in our own hotel, a seasonal game feast in the dining room: a wunderbar menu and extravagant decorations of mounted partridge and hare and deer. The hotel chef owned a forest, and each year he produced a week-long game gala.

"I really won't be going off my diet if I skip the sauces. Game is absolutely free of fat," I told Bill. "I won't have any wine or even a drop of German beer. We can manage."

It was a memorable week. We stored enjoyment for the future the way you charge a battery. And the game was delicious: partridge, hare, pheasant, venison.

By the middle of the first week most of the people at our hotel knew that I intended to check in at the Janker Klinik. The treatment was a major topic of gossip and innuendo, much of it from our host, the hotel manager. He told us that many Janker patients had stayed at the hotel before beginning treatment, and sometimes afterward—although by then they were listless, emaciated shadows, too weak to do more than leave for home on a stretcher. He said that some patients were driven literally mad during the aftermath of the drugs.

For months, six months certainly, my right ankle and foot had been traumatized by a series of recurring sprains. Once or twice I had torn ligaments there. At first the swelling would go down between mishaps, but later it refused; the edema became permanent, no matter how many times I tried the whirlpool bath. I elevated my foot faithfully for hours, but the condition persisted until my doctors in New York could only dismiss it as "something that will have to heal itself." Instead of healing, there had been deterioration: walking was occasionally quite painful, the cane increasingly necessary, and I realized by the numbness in the area that my circulation was very poor. Still I walked—or limped—determinedly, but it was a real relief to learn as I came in for my first cobalt treatment at Janker that Dr. Hoefer had left orders that I was also to receive circulation therapy for my foot. Apparently he could notice something about a patient besides cancerous tumors! In New York, I often had the distinct impression that I appeared to all my doctors simply as a disembodied Cancerous Lung and that any other disability was too secondary to merit consideration. In Bonn, Dr. Hoefer explained that the poor circulation in my right foot was not merely an unfortunate aftermath of repeated injuries but a common side effect of radiation therapy. The closing of fragile capillaries and consequent shutting-off of the flow of blood to the extremities of cancer patients who had had deep radiation was often seen, he said. I was glad of the explanation and wondered why no doctor in New York had even hinted at that.

The circulation therapy I was given at Janker consisted of four wide tapes of feltlike material wrapped around my right leg from ankle to thigh. The tapes were connected by tubes to a machine whose pumping action expanded and contracted them in sequence, mimicking the flow of natural circulation and at the same time massaging the affected parts. After the second treatment, though my foot was still swollen, I was nevertheless able to walk back to the hotel without my cane. It was a victory and this small event, this concern about my total health shown by Dr. Hoefer, helped to steady me as the week of grace ended. At the hotel, the manager now revealed his total belief that the Janker treatment could add years to the life of a cancer patient and he confessed that he himself had cancer of the colon and was planning to "do something about it," check in at Janker, as soon as he could "find the courage." I now understood his obsession with horror stories.

The day came up gray, drizzling and chill. My foot had improved enough so that I walked to the Klinik with Bill. We didn't talk much. There is no way to say "Death is snapping at my heels again, perhaps torture can stay it" without cracking the thin, precious shell of calm. So we walked and felt and ached and hoped—silently. The Klinik was in full swing when we arrived, the rattling old elevator going down to the cellar where the cobalt treatments were given, the stolid nurses, the darting technicians, the lines of outpatients lengthening in the waiting room. But this time we went up instead of down, directly to my assigned room on the third floor. The room was mostly ceiling; its compass very small. Bed, couch, table and armoire crowded it to the walls. A nurse was waiting for me, the only nurse for the six rooms on my floor. She was a flinty-eyed veteran as belligerent as a hose-sprayed wasp. When we showed surprise at the tiny room, she took it as an insult toward the whole Janker Klinik. The rooms on the first and second floors were enormous, she informed us. The Klinik had one hundred and ten beds, did we realize that? But it did not have the luxury of big grants from the government or private foundations such as all American hospitals could have for the asking. Yet it had a greater reputation for saving cancer patients than most American hospitals. But something more serious than good personal relations was missing from my room, and Bill was the first to say so. "Where's the bathroom?" he asked. "At the end of the hall," said my Florence Nightingale. "It is shared." Shared? There were six rooms on the floor; that meant six patients and the nurse. Suddenly Bill and I were homesick for the privacy of plumbing that Americans take for granted. In my case, a communal bathroom at the end of the hall could be a disaster. How would I manage to get there if I had a drastic reaction to the chemotherapy? I closed my eyes, remembering the dreadful diarrhea, the complete loss of control that had wracked me after the sessions in New York. What if it happened again? What if the shared bathroom was occupied at the critical moment? Bill, reading my face, said, "Just don't worry about it. We'll manage somehow."

As the nurse began to unpack my clothes she suddenly spoke to Bill. "I suppose you were in Germany during the war?" Startled, he said no. "During the occupation?" she persisted. "No," said Bill. "This is my first visit to Germany." But she seemed skeptical. I could imagine her forming more questions to test us, to bait us into apologizing for being Americans. We tried to redirect the conversation, but she brought it back to the same subject. And when she hung away my fur coat, she stroked it and said, "Is it true that American women will wear only mink?" I decided that I'd had enough of this treatment. My instincts told me that I must put an end to the bullying, so I pitched my voice to parade-ground level and answered her rudeness. "Nurse, we have come here on far more important business than to listen to such chatter as this. The sooner we get down to the details of my routine, the better."

There was silence: when she spoke again it was in an entirely different voice. Her words were courteous. Perhaps she realized that the war was over and her personal losses were thirty years in the past. Perhaps she realized that I wouldn't let her bully me even though I was vulnerable and dependent on her services. I don't know why, but from that day on she treated me with exaggerated courtesy. I had no cause for complaint. She was a good nurse. I even came to like her and she—begrudgingly— even got to like me.

The Janker Klinik was profoundly Teutonic. We were still unpacking that first morning when we heard what seemed to be a light troop of soldiers draw up sharply in the hall outside in perfect synchronization. There was a brusque knock and the door swung open to admit Dr. Hoefer and a parade of associates and assistants. "Parade" was the only possible description. They all wished us "Guten Morgen" and they all lined up shoulder to shoulder, clipboards at the ready, white coats blinding in their crisp perfection and Dr. Hoefer's far outdazzling the rest. No one lounged, no one slouched and, alas, no one smiled. But even in the dazzling-white paramilitary atmosphere, I could feel Dr. Hoefer's kindness. I could sense the compassion that drove him to begin his work at five in the morning and kept him working until late at night; trying to see one more desperate patient, make one more diagnosis, take in one more cancer case.

Today's visit had the purpose of formally presenting us to the medical staff of the Janker Klinik and explaining the procedure of the Trophosphamide therapy I would experience. Dr. Scheef, the Chief of Staff, was there and also a bearded young doctor who was in daily charge, the floor doctor. He would be responsible for my daily routines, for the entries on my chart and the general report on my condition. Bill was especially anxious to make personal contact with this "man on the spot" and he shook hands with him immediately. (You can't go wrong shaking hands in a Teutonic society; the difficulty is in knowing when to stop.)

Now Dr. Hoefer began to explain what would happen tomorrow, the day that I would receive the first of two infusions of Trophosphamide. In the morning the nurse would bring me eight large capsules to be taken at specific intervals between 7 A.M. and 10 A.M. At 10:30 the infusion would begin and it would last the standard three hours, until 1:30 in the afternoon. Immediately after that, I must begin to counter the deleterious effects of Trophosphamide by consuming quarts and quarts of liquids. The first quart must be Fachinger water, a bottled mineral water that immediately flushes the kidneys. After that I could take fruit juices and tea—but I must keep drinking for twenty-four hours. There could be no letup, no periods of undisturbed sleep. It was literally a case of drinking to live, drinking to keep liquid flowing through the kidneys, washing out the deadly residue to Trophosphamide or risking death by kidney failure. The very extreme concentration of the drug had to be countered by constant liquid intake and output of urine. Urination was life, quite literally, and lack of it was death, so precise records must be kept of the amount of liquid going in and the amount of urine being excreted. I would have a two-liter beaker, graded on a scale of 100 to 2,000 grams, with which to measure my output. I must keep this record for twenty-four hours, and it would be repeated the next day, after the second infusion.

My first thought when the doctor finished speaking was of the distance down the hall to the communal bathroom. If anyone needed to be assigned the highest priority for emergency use, it would be I, shuttling between bedroom and bathroom with measuring beaker in hand. But others had done it; I could do it as well. I thought of my newest X-rays—and shuddered. I had all the incentive I needed.

In the morning I bathed in the communal tub and made myself ready by 7 A.M. At 7:05, Bill arrived with a satchel of fresh oranges and an orange squeezer he had bought in the town square. As he did every day, he made me a large glass of fresh orange juice. Then he laid out a dozen super-size bottles of assorted fruit juices. He had brought graph paper and pens; together we made out our own charts listing Intake, Output and Time. The nurse brought my eight capsules and I took the first with the orange juice. The infusion was three and a quarter hours away. Bill had done everything he could; now I began to prepare in my own way, to rehearse mentally, to do it all in advance, willing what I wanted to happen, willing success.

At 10:30, when the infusion began, I thought that everything was under control. But shortly afterward, a familiar nausea began to rise until I was choking and gagging, eyes streaming with fluids. Why weren't my nausea suppressants working? I soon found out—I hadn't been given any! The day before I'd told the nurse that I had a bad reaction to Compozine and could not have it as a suppressant prior to my infusion. Through the considerable language barrier, she'd understood me to say that I was allergic to suppressants and should be given none. But I must have some relief quickly or I would be too ravaged by cramps to drink even one glass of life-saving liquid. After several hysterical moments, the nurse pounded off in search of the floor doctor. As soon as the doctor came, he gave me a shot and my stomach quieted almost immediately. My mouth opened to breathe again, my fists unclenched, my back relaxed. The chemical was still going in, but I knew it was downhill all the way now. Somehow this Trophosphamide produced none of the raging aftereffects of the chemotherapy I had known before. Afterward, I was able to make normal trips to the end of the hall without the desperate diarrheic sprinting I remembered. Strange, for this was far more potent poison than the mustard-gas derivatives I had taken in New York.

By 2 A.M. I was rewarded for my massive "drinking bout." Our charts showed an encouraging output of 2,000 grams. By dawn, it was an intake of 3,000 and an output of 3,250. I realized that I was getting through it with only half the expected effort. And there wasn't that intolerable pain, that feeling of every fiber of me splitting that I associated with chemotherapy. Perhaps the continuous flushing of the kidneys had spared me. The time ticked away. I drank obediently . . . it was morning and then noon and then the afternoon of the second infusion. Night . . . dawn . . . morning . . . and still I was more than holding my own. Finally, I took my last drink. I lay back, breathing shallowly, letting my mind drift away from the fierce knot of concentration, the fist I had made of it. The danger of kidney failure was over. And now I could only wait, wait through the critical ten-day period after the infusions. The battle was inside me now, raging in my blood.

"You realize that your white-cell blood count will be danger-ously low," Dr. Hoefer had said to me. "It will go below a thousand, probably as low as three hundred. But not at once, of course. The count begins to drop after four or five days, and then, on the tenth day, it will reach its lowest point."

And then?

"And then," the doctor said, "you must be very, very careful to avoid infection. During the period that your white-cell blood count is below one thousand you will have lost your resistance and even a mild infection could be fatal."

How could I, lying in a hospital bed, prevent infection from entering my room? "What do you suggest?" I'd asked. "Should I station my husband at the door to stop anyone who coughs or sneezes from coming into my room?"

The intended irony went unnoticed.

"Those are good procedures, Mrs. McGrail," said the doctor. And he turned to Bill. "You had better avoid crowds at the hotel. Don't take the elevator, don't hesitate to leave a room if anyone sneezes or coughs. Your wife will be dangerously vulnerable and you are coming to see her every day. If you yourself feel the slightest bit unwell, don't come."

But Bill had no intention of leaving me alone. I needed his help. I could not do without that help. I think he may have saved my life several times during the infusions—and now he arrived every morning at seven after an invariable early breakfast of coffee and boiled eggs. He still brought fresh oranges and squeezed juice for me, but now we scrubbed the oranges with hot water first to try to eliminate any possible cold germ that might contaminate them. The thought of the food trays from the Klinik kitchen frightened me. I couldn't afford not to eat for days, but I wondered who down in the kitchen had a cold, who coughed as my tray went by, who had children sick with influenza at home and came to work because he or she couldn't afford to lose the day's wages. I wondered if any special measures were being taken to protect my food from casual contamination. Somehow, I doubted it. The Germans had a rough-and-ready attitude. There was a category of risk they obviously found acceptable and they seemed to hold the patient responsible for his own safety. I would think wistfully of our American obsession with anti-germ sprays, constant disinfectants, disposable hypodermics and disposable sheets in our hospitals. But I was here in Germany because our germ-conscious hospitals at home could do nothing more to help me. I had to be here, had to take my chances. I was at the mercy of anyone's sneeze, anyone's slightly rheumy eye, cough, spittle, infected cut. What was merely a nuisance to someone else could take my life now. The woman who cleaned my room each day had a strange-looking rash on her hands—I would ask her not to come. Every night I heard coughing in the hall. And I already felt a tightening in my chest each time someone knocked at my door. It was panic. Now I knew how paranoia could develop. And I still had days to go!

# CHAPTER XIV

# Hans and Fritz in Bonn

One week after my Trophosphamide infusion, with my white-cell blood count declining from 5,600 to a still safe 2,300, I had put that first paranoia behind me. The time had not yet come when I'd be a prisoner in my room; I could still go to X-ray to check on the Trophosphamide's effect on my tumor and also be examined by a specialist who was coming from Munich to look at my sightless eye. It was a period of grace, of anticipatory hope, and I was so anxious to know the results of the X-rays I had had taken that I questioned the floor doctor, Dr. Zilkin, whose understanding of English was not nearly as good as he imagined.

"Doctor, have you seen my X-rays?"

He nodded. "Ja."

"Has there been a change?"

He began to struggle for the right English word.

"The tumor is—ah . . ."

"Shrunk?" I supplied helpfully.

"Shrunk. Ja, ja, very good. The tumor is shrunk."

It sounded good, especially when I was taken off cobalt later that day. The next morning, Dr. Hoefer made his official visit and I was eager to hear his report.

"Doctor, what did the X-rays show?"

He smiled. "The tumor has disappeared."

"Shrunk" or "disappeared"? I couldn't account for the discrepancy. Bill suggested that I might have myself to blame: I had supplied the floor doctor with "shrunk" and he might only have guessed at its meaning. Dr. Hoefer, in spite of his difficult English, had not groped, had spoken precisely.

"Let's believe Dr. Hoefer's version," Bill said.

And so we did, until the next morning, when my discontinued cobalt treatments began again without explanation. "Shrunk" or "disappeared"? The uncertainty remained.

Time after time we were daunted by apparent inconsistencies. One treatment was given to "stabilize" another which we had understood was conclusive; adjunct therapies started and stopped, doctors seemed sometimes to contradict each other. We realized it was all due to the language barrier, but in defense, to encourage each other, Bill and I began to call ourselves Hans and Fritz in Bonn. We never did it when the German staff could overhear and perhaps misunderstand: Hans and Fritz was our private code for "Hang in there." It was an amusing little thing at first—Hans and Fritz, the original Katzenjammer Kids, everything happened to them. But gradually, Hans and Fritz became a lifeline, a way of looking at things, a way of solving the problems that arose from our surroundings and somehow extracting a little fun wherever and whenever it was possible to do so. Hans and Fritz made end runs around the opposition, Hans and Fritz brought the outside world to the inside room: *they* were not shackled to cancer, they were free.

One of the problems Hans and Fritz had to solve was the Klinik menu. I had expected to be able to continue on my

Freund diet; this was Germany, after all, this was where Doctor Freund had done much of his research. But virtually everything on my lunch tray was forbidden: thick slabs of bread still warm from the kitchen oven, accompanied by an earthen crock of sweet butter. The Freund diet banned yeast products of all kinds and butter was strictly forbidden. I remembered the taste of bread longingly, the memory swung like a pendulum between Irish soda bread slathered in butter, the wonderful Easter loaves of my childhood, the best white bread I had ever eaten—in Bombay. I wanted to dive at this temptation, to scoop mounds of butter on the fragrant slices but I asked Bill to take the breadbasket off my tray and out of the room.

Then I lifted the cover on the main course. There was fresh cauliflower à la Polonaise, boiled potato dripping in melted butter and a piece of succulent roast pork edged on all sides with crisp fat. *Verboten*, all specifically forbidden to me. I had no intention of negating those months of discipline I had come through for bread, fat pork and cauliflower. If this was the Klinik food, if the Freund diet was not only not followed but absolutely defied, what would I eat? Hans and Fritz would have to think of something.

Dr. Hoefer admitted that he was familiar with the Freund diet and believed it effective but he could not use it at the Klinik. The reason was, the patients, a cross-section of the German population "Are used to basic foods. Ninety percent of the world's population subsists on the food Dr. Freund forbids. If we told patients that they had to give up bread and butter and cheese and cabbage, these people would find it impossible to be treated for cancer. We would be limiting help for just too many."

I couldn't help feeling that if there was a reasonable chance of a cancer cure or cancer deterrent in nutritional therapy, then it should be pursued regardless of obstacles. Freund had done it with his Austrian peasants at severe sacrifice to them. And nutrition would certainly be a gentle adjunct to the brutal ravages of chemotherapy and radiotherapy. But I knew the arguments on the medical side—standard cancer treatment takes comparatively little time, it's easier to control, and it can be evaluated with X-rays anywhere in the world. I suppose that was Dr. Hoefer's real answer. Cancer is so terrifying that we opt for drastic measures. A simpler, more natural, a more subtle approach is not honored as a treatment or even as an adjunct to treatment.

Still, I would not eat most Klinik meals, although it was wonderful Middle European home cooking. Bill—who was usually Frizt—decided to be my supplier. He knew the Bonn market plaza and the inventories of the little shops around it so well by this time that he was able to buy fresh chickens and fish for me and have them cooked in the Klinik kitchen. He found the only store in Bonn that carried Irish oatmeal and brought it to the cooks. I don't know what they thought; it was definitely not the German breakfast, which leans heavily to cold cuts, sliced cheeses, mounds of bread and coffee, but under Bill's direction, they began to make Irish oatmeal for me. Sometimes Bill slipped down to the kitchen and made up batches in advance which then needed only reheating. The kitchen became so accommodating in so many little ways—no butter on my vegetables, salad at lunch and dinner—that I knew Bill had been dispensing Deutschmarks in his usual liberal vein. But I was back on a good approximation of the Freund diet and I believed it would give me the stamina to come through these treatments with my nerves intact.

So Hans and Fritz became a daily supply operation as well as a motto of endurance. I had my appointment with the Munich eye specialist. He was not encouraged by my medical history, especially the radiation, and when, after the examination, I asked if I would ever see with that eye again, he answered, "Never, the retina and optic nerve have been destroyed."

To begin with, the tumor in my eye was not a "freak." Janker Klinik doctors often saw such a metastasis to the eye in patients with lung cancer and breast cancer. They were able to treat it: radiate the tumor and restore some degree of sight. But I had had massive radiation to the eye in New York. At Janker Klinik, working with far smaller amounts of radiation, they considered a figure of a thousand rads as "overkill." The three thousand I had taken in New York had burned out my retina. There was no hope of regaining sight.

"You have no sign of a brain tumor," the Munich specialist told me. I replied that I hadn't thought of a brain tumor. "But it can easily happen in lung cancer metastasis," he said. "Oh, then perhaps that is why my New York doctors, in their anxiety to prevent a brain tumor, had given me the extra dose of radiation that destroyed my eye," I reasoned.

Hans and Fritz worked harder after that at producing diversions. We were almost completely isolated from the life around us by the language barrier. Just once a day the radio carried a program with two or three items about Great Britain delivered in impeccable Oxford English. We waited for that. There was a daily edition of the overseas *Herald Tribune*: Bill bought it every morning and we read it item by item all day long. The only magazine available in English was *Newsweek* and we devoured every word. In desperation, I called the American Embassy in Bonn, asking for back-issues magazines. Bill began a daily vigil at the hotel mail desk and for seven days there was nothing—nothing until, at a time when my blood count had dipped below the danger line, the magazines finally arrived. But I never saw them. They were so soiled, grease-marked and unsanitary that Bill tossed them into a trash basket as soon as he opened the package. It was an unbelievable disappointment. Outside the weather held winter-gray and chilling; inside, perhaps because they missed the sun, the serious people around us rarely smiled.

To pass the time, we made daily rituals, formalizing each activity as if civilization depended on these small ceremonies. There was the Squeezing of the Orange Juice when Bill arrived each morning at 7:30; a golden flow of substitute sunlight except for the morning when he brought Sicilian oranges whose blood-red juice I refused because it made me feel like Dracula. There was the Ritual of the Surprise, the mystery of what Bill might bring back from his daily ten o'clock run to the stores and stalls of the market plaza. He'd bring fresh food for my diet, of course, and always fruit, which we chilled on the tiny, cracked balcony ledge outside my window. Sometimes it was pure wool panty hose and those wonderful European woolen camisoles and leggings; other times superb Puma budding knives for summer gardening activites. And flowers—I remember anemones and a double armload of freesias that blazed like Riviera sunshine in the room. One day he surpassed himself; I think it was the day after the specialist told me that my eye was ruined. Bill arrived with a delicate wicker basket. In the basket, on a bed of the tiny, growing curled mustard greens used to top salads, sat a marzipan frog, green as pond lilies and wearing a gold paper crown.

I didn't realize that the doctors were watching our Hans and Fritz activities. But they marked Bill's attendance each morning, noticed how he came back after lunch and lingered through the Ritual of Reading the Paper until late afternoon when he left for his solitary swim, sauna and dinner at the hotel. I am sure they did not understand the rituals, the special foods, the gifts which delighted us both. How could they? They were at home; we were the foreigners. But they conferred and came to the

Teutonic conclusion that Bill was suffering from an over-developed sense of duty. Dr. Hoefer began to hint to me that Bill would be better off in New York.

There was no need for both of us to wait out my treatment, he said. Wouldn't I feel better knowing that Mr. McGrail was living his normal life? And what about his business?

What they couldn't know was that our normal life was being together, in business and after hours. We had chosen each other in second marriages because we wanted to share our lives completely. Together we built a joint design for living. For me, Bill had changed from a double martini drinker to a moderate connoisseur of wines. For him, I had learned to shoot game and wade in icy trout streams. For each other we gardened, pampered our cats, traveled, built our country place with love and imagination, timber by antique timber, gambrel, gable and patchwork quilt. Our life was each other and now my misfortune had drawn us defensively closer. Even our Hans and Fritz identities were interchangeable.

Bill fielded the doctors' hints that he should go home; all he needed to do business, he said, was a long-distance telephone. These were brave words and we stood firm. But then a telephone call made us realize how much we needed contact with our own family, our own world. The day before my blood count was expected to plummet to its lowest, Bill's sister Jean called to say that she was in Germany on a trip and could she come to visit us in Bonn? Now I could understand what a family visit means to a shut-in; we could barely wait for Jean to bring New York to us! I wouldn't be able to see her until my count rose, of course, but it would be nice that she would be at Bill's dinner table each evening, that Bill could take her meandering through the old plaza. "Pray that she doesn't have a cold," I said. If she did then Bill couldn't see her either, because I was so vulnerable.

But Jean arrived intact from the healthy world bringing English magazines and a blessed paperback. She was renewal therapy for Bill; and I began to count time again. In sixteen days the doctors had said that my white-cell blood count would be at near-normal. After that, we might make plans to go home. Home—if nothing else happened. But the next morning, a sunny morning for Bonn, Dr. Zilkin appeared in the doorway with the nurse and a chemotherapy rack.

"Today," said the doctor, "you will receive a special infusion. It will help to make ze cobalt more effective. But remember, you must be careful to avoid fever."

This mysterious announcement was entirely typical. One morning the same Doctor Zilkin had come rushing into my room to say, "Cobalt stops. You are overradiated." We panicked until we discovered that the message had gained something in translation: all the doctor meant to say was that I had finished the scheduled course of cobalt treatments.

I never did understand my schedule; it was stop-and-go all the way. First, no more cobalt, then suddenly, five more cobalts, and then, before I could comply, cobalt was cancelled again. Now, today, there was a mysterious infusion to help "ze cobalt." And the warning to avoid fever. For the hundredth time I wished that we had brought someone who could speak German with us, someone to interpret both the treatment and the doctors.

Dr. Zilkin indicated that he wanted to get on with the infusion.

"Are there side effects?" I hedged.

"Only stomachitis."

"And how would I know if I developed that?"

"Zere would come sores in the mouth. Zat would be bad."

"Would these sores come right away?"

"Oh, no, not so soon. Perhaps after ze tenth infusion."

When I heard that, I shrieked. I couldn't help it.

Ten infusions! At Columbia Presbyterian, one chemotherapy infusion every six weeks was an exercise in stoicism. Now I faced one a day for ten days, an adjunct to the Trophosphamide, to sensitize the tissue exposed to cobalt. But no one had mentioned ten new infusions to me; the chemotherapy rack had simply appeared in my room.

"Bill, I can't do it." I meant it; I desperately wanted to get out of there, race to the airport, fly out of the country. Vanish.

"We've gone this far . . ." But Bill looked as if he wanted to run with me.

"We'll call Dr. Hoefer—straighten this out." Bill was up and pacing, close to blowup, I knew.

"Dr. Hoefer ordered ze infusions," the floor doctor said.

"I want to talk to him!"

For the first time, I saw Bill near a breaking point. Before this, he had always managed to put a good face on things and rally me, but this last "surprise" had shaken him completely.

"If Dr. Hoefer's ordered it, what's the sense of fighting?" I reasoned numbly. "As you said, we've come this far."

All I knew was that if Bill gave in to nervous despondency, my own control would disappear. We decided to go ahead.

The first infusion—"It will be three hours," I was told—lasted for four and a half hours. No explanation. And I finished it in a state of semi-paralysis: the nurse had forgotten to put a supporting board under my arm, and I lay rigid, not daring to move that arm once the flow had begun. Afterward, I was really angry but it didn't help. "Oh, ja," said the nurse. "Oh, ja, we use the board tomorrow."

The infusion did not make me feel unwell, and so I was considerably calmer at the second one. When I brushed my teeth that night, I noticed some small swellings on my inner lips; they were painless, exactly the sort of thing you might get if you bit your lips in angry frustration. On the morning of the third infusion, I mentioned them to Dr. Zilkin.

"You drink too much orange juice," he said. "Every morning, orange juice. It makes acid."

Dr. Scheef, the Klinik director, appeared in the doorway. I hadn't seen him for a while. He was always on the run, always trailing reassurances as he sped away from you—privately Bill and I called him the Electrified Cat.

Today he was mellow and had time to examine me. He made pleasant conversation in English, asked me some questions and looked closely into my mouth. Suddenly, staccato German burst like machine-gun fire in Dr. Zilkin's direction. Dr. Zilkin answered, disagreeing, standing his ground. But Dr. Scheef looked furious.

"I am discontinuing the infusions!"

To me, he explained that the little lumps I'd seen were the warning "sores," appearing days ahead of schedule as unmistakable evidence that my body was reacting unfavorably to the infusions. "I am ordering antibiotics for you. You must take them at once. And every hour, I want you to gargle with camomile tea. Every hour!"

For once he did not tell me how well I was doing. And the infusions were not reinstated, apparently for good reason. Some particular Providence had sent the busy, brilliant Dr. Scheef into my room on that particular day, perhaps saving my life.

In the midst of all this my white-cell blood count began to recover and edge upward. The doctors had said that it would, but in my current understandable state of confusion, I had to see the numbers for myself. Each day the technician took a blood sample and the results were available from the laboratory after two o'clock. My lowest level was 500, then it rose to 700, and two days later to 1,500. As it edged toward 2,000, Bill produced optimism from the depths of his gloom like a magician bringing out a rabbit. Perhaps, he temporized, we were too accustomed to the niceties of Harkness Pavilion and to doctors who had time to explain their procedures. These busy, overworked people dashing through the halls didn't have time to do it our way.

"Look," said Bill. "Maybe we should stop reacting to inconveniences and decide if we want you saved or whether you have to be saved with class."

Both Hans and Fritz found that very funny.

The next day my count had reached the point where it was safe for me to walk in the hall outside my room, resuming the exercise period I'd taken daily at the beginning of my Janker Klinik stay. Bill walked with me—it was a way to walk the edge off his restlessness—and I persevered out of sheer pleasure at the improvement in my foot. It was so good to fit it into a shoe again! But I went carefully, never resting my full weight on the weak side, always trying to compensate with my stronger foot. As we shuffled along together, our conversations took a hopeful turn: when this is over, when we go home— Day by day, the time of my discharge was growing nearer.

When I closed my eyes each night I saw the streets of New York as they looked from the living room of our apartment, light streaming through the green jungle of plants we had turned toward the morning sun. I missed that room and I especially missed the two fat city cats who loved to lounge in the morning sunlight.

It was strange for me to be living a "catless" life. My first feeling of uneasiness driving through Bonn had been the uncanny absence of cats: no cats sitting in the windows, none on the streets, not even a cat near the fish market. For two who love felines as thoroughly and personally as Bill and I do, their absence was a deprivation and a mystery. Everywhere else in the world we had seen cats: here were dogs, well-trained, well-fed dogs, and box turtles in pet shops (they're believed to be lucky), but no cats. One day Bill found out why. In Bonn, cats were in demand as Katzenfelds, cat skins used to treat the aches and pains of rheumatism and arthritis. They were sold as complete skinned cat furs—folded flat, packed in little boxes with pictures of smiling kitties on them and available in drugstores. When Bill told me that he saw the Katzenfelds in drugstore windows, I didn't believe him. The nurse confirmed it. "Ja," she said. "We use Katzenfelds for rheumatism." I wanted to throw bricks through all the windows of all the drugstores in Bonn. In my mind I began composing rash, indignant letters to Chancellor Helmut Schmidt: what a shame that little German children would never know the joy of snuggling a soft, purring kitten instead of meeting it as a poultice on Grandfather's rheumatic hip.

The day that I was discharged from the Janker Klinik the sun made one of its rare appearances. I walked through the front door, past the brass plate and out onto the boulevard, well bundled in fur coat and sturdy shoes. The first breath of outside air pierced my lungs and when I looked at the snowy line of trees, witnesses to my survival, a sudden weakness made them swim in circles till the vertiginous moment passed. I was weak in a way I could never have imagined; not lacking strength to lift my hands and feet but weak from within, hollow, empty, scooped out. The chemicals that killed cancer cells had taken my substance, too. All that was left of me was a shell held together by memory and faintly quivering nerves. I was almost invisible to myself, almost transparent to the feeble sun—and this was the cure I had fought to attain. It had sucked the marrow of my bones like a greedy giant. At the slightest touch I felt that I might scatter on the wind.

I had told Bill earlier that I wanted to walk the block and a half to the hotel, and so I did. Putting down one foot and then the other, seeing my footprints in the snow made me feel less invisible, reaffirmed my existence . . . and I was walking away from the Klinik. There would be only one farewell meeting, a conference with Dr. Hoefer, and then, that same day, we'd step on the plane to New York. As I walked, I imagined happier times: I conjured up our country house with its sleeping gardens and winter-fluffed cats and next summer's flowers under the snow. My old pride had crept back into me by the time we reached the hotel steps. I looked up and had a sudden vision of myself mounting the steps as I had before the days of the traumatized foot, one proud foot in front of the other. If I could do it again, it would be a sign that one day my energy would flow back into my body; one day I would not only walk but dance again. I set my strong foot on the first step, swung up the weaker to the second step, leaned forward just a little too much! With a crunching sound—quite audible—my right foot twisted under me and I staggered back against Bill, who was coming up behind me. I didn't need the sudden spurt of pain to tell me what had happened. I knew. I had sprained it, all over again.

So it was with definite déjà vu, just like the morning that we arrived, that I sat in Dr. Hoefer's office with cane and swollen foot. He was properly sympathetic but felt that the general condition of my foot had improved and suggested that I talk to the doctors in New York about circulation therapy.

I said that I was anxious to do that.

We looked at each other. After a somewhat tentative pause, Bill asked Dr. Hoefer for a personal evaluation of my general condition, a guideline we ourselves could follow.

"Mrs. McGrail's condition," said the doctor, "is satisfactory."

Satisfactory?

The lukewarm, cautious word dismayed us both. Its narrow compass suggested failure.

"Oh, not at all." Dr. Hoefer seemed surprised by our reaction. "Mrs. McGrail, your condition is indeed satisfactory but it is in the next round of treatments that you will see a really dramatic improvement."

A frozen silence. Bill asked incredulously, "What was that, Doctor?"

Dr. Hoefer repeated it, adding, "You have completed the first part of our two-part therapy. You go home now and we will expect to see Mrs. McGrail back here in six weeks. Then we begin again."

This was the first time a two-part therapy had been mentioned. I had never heard of it before but I refused to consider it for one moment.

"Doctor Hoefer, I will not be coming back."

He explained that my chances for a prolonged remission and possible recovery almost doubled during the second round of treatments.

How could a kind man like Dr. Hoefer have saved this thunderbolt for last and in one sentence taken away my joy, my illusion of freedom? I was sustained only by the idea that it was all over, that I was finished with treatments for a long time to come—perhaps forever. That was all that held my shreds and pieces together. But now . . . I looked at Bill, silently pleading: Let's get out of here.

Bill wanted to know just how much difference the second round of treatments would make.

Dr. Hoefer answered that a certain level of remission was reached after the first six weeks of treatment but that their statistics proved that the second six weeks produced a remission of much longer duration, a remission that could extend to many years—even recovery became a possibility. And the finale of this second six weeks was a series of white-cell immunology injections that would stimulate my own immunology, increase my white-cell count still further, and bring back the resistance and the strength I had lost. I would not feel then as I did now.

"Why can't I take the next six weeks series in New York—perhaps you or Dr. Scheef can fly over."

It seemed that there were many reasons. The Trophosphamide treatment was not recognized in the United States so it could not be given in a hospital. Where then would I take it? How would I counter the unfavorable side effects, the kidney dysfunction? No, it was impossible. Even with a doctor they knew, a former Janker associate now working in New York, it was entirely too dangerous. And it was illegal. And the cobalt could not be administered outside a hospital. Altogether, it would not be possible. Only at the Klinik could it be totally controlled.

I heard Bill say, "All right. In six weeks we'll be back."

"Bill!"

He didn't want to look at me. I wondered if I was crying, whether my tears had surfaced. Inside me a candle was flickering, and it might go out at any time. The worst six weeks of my life were to be repeated. I had no strength to argue, but I did not think that I would survive another cure.

At the hotel, as he packed for me, I saw Bill slip a flat long strip of metal into my suitcase. It was a German license plate, a Bonn automobile license plate. Black letters on a white background. But it had no numbers. Instead, it said: HANS UND FRITZ IN BONN.

Bill, watching my face, said, "Sorry about the 'und.' I wanted 'and' but the man who made it didn't get the idea."

"Where did you get it?" I asked and was amazed that I was still capable of giggling with delight.

"It's your diploma; you're graduated with honors," Bill said proudly.

"Our diploma," I corrected.

I will always remember, when I look at the whimsical license plate, how it was and how Hans and Fritz endured it together.

# CHAPTER XV

# Thirteen Golden Needles

In early March of 1976 I felt that I had finally won a respite from cancer. There was no sign of malignancy, and two dry-cell immunological injections would be administered to me in New York to keep my own body defenses working against the disease. After the second round of Trophosphamide therapy in Bonn, I had my first dry-cell immunological injection and my white-cell blood count had risen from its low of 500 to 6,200—600 points higher than it had been even prior to surgery.

Dr. Stock's reaction seemed to oscillate between delight and disbelief. I knew that he could not bring himself to make a connection between my startling improvement and Janker Klinik: Janker, which used drugs still illegal in America, which allowed a patient's blood count to drop to lethal levels and then pushed new drug therapy on the supposed corpse. This was not Dr. Stock's idea of correct procedures. When I had staggered into his office after the first round of Janker treatments, Dr. Stock had shouted at me like a despairing parent: "The Germans did this to you! You look dreadful! Why did you have to go there?"

Now here I was again, vitality renewed, blood count soaring and optimism matching it. Dr. Stock examined me carefully. He found everything fine, except the maddening right foot, which had not responded as well to the second round of circulation therapy. It was stiff and wooden, unmanageable, always cold, and it dragged behind me like a stranger. I told Dr. Stock that it had been tested for cancer in Germany; he nodded, but made an immediate appointment with the orthopedic specialist at Columbia Presbyterian.

There was another cancer test, and another negative answer. Then there was an orthopedic diagnosis: my problem was that I had forgotten how to walk! During all of the months of repeated injuries to that right foot, I had lost my gait, lost the ability to walk properly, and because of the inevitable dragging I now had a severe calcium deficiency in the bones of my right foot. This, combined with the very poor circulation due to shrunken capillaries—a by-product of heavy radiation, Dr. Hoefer had explained—had left me with a traumatized foot that needed serious, constant therapy.

The orthopedic specialist recommended a physical doctor affiliated with Columbia Presbyterian, whose field of expertise was orthopedic therapy. His office was only a block from our apartment but I still had to take a taxi to get there. Hobbling down the block with what looked like a drunken sailor's lurch was embarrassing and painful. Even our cats in the country fled when they saw me dragging toward them.

I used a cane, I went faithfully to the physical doctor's therapist for treatment three times a week, and I bought a whirlpool bath for home use. Nothing helped very much. After each excruciatingly painful manipulation by the therapist, my foot would swell to the ankle, as shapeless as a child's football. Shoes and slippers were out of the question; I wore an improvised cloth boot. It didn't keep my foot warm: nothing warmed my frigid foot that mild, sunny April. I sat with my bulbous foot swathed in a heavy woolen sock and an electric heating pad.

The therapist thought I might see progress in six months; I asked about some other method of treatment. Dr. Yu, the physical doctor, was licensed to practice acupuncture and after considering my plight, he announced that we would try it. I was immediately hopeful. The papers had recently carried almost daily accounts of acupuncture wonder cures. Acupuncture had raised the hopes of every sufferer from chronic pain, so my only question to the doctor was "When?"

In two weeks, he told me. I reported jubilantly to Bill. "Won't it be wonderful not to be plagued with this foot?"

"It hasn't happened yet," Bill replied reasonably.

I liked the premise of acupuncture: no drugs, no radiation, an ages-old technique using the body's nervous system to block the gateways to pain.

My enthusiasm finally reached Bill and he decided to take the treatment himself to alleviate a persistent stinging in his left big toe. Dr. Yu said that Bill could be helped but warned that the sole of the foot was perhaps the only truly painful area for acupuncture. "I have seen big strong men faint when acupuncture was performed on the sole of the foot."

But Bill replied: "When Joie has her sessions, I'll take mine. Don't worry about me fainting."

Bill was in the waiting room as I lay on the table in the acupuncturist's office. I was fascinated by Dr. Yu's long golden needles, poetically slender and shimmering . . . I thought of dragonflies. First he told me that there would be thirteen placements of the needles beginning at my calf down to my ankle and instep. I nodded, smiled—it would be painless so I didn't brace myself.

The shock and agonizing pain that followed proved beyond

my endurance. I heard my voice screaming to crescendoes as every needle jabbed into my flesh. The room echoed with my involuntary screams, like a madhouse. When the needles were all placed, the pain began to ebb. Heart thudding, I wondered what could have happened? Why this indescribable pain? It was supposed to be painless.

The doctor remained unperturbed, making only indirect reference to my screams by saying that he'd better go out and reassure Bill. "I will return in twenty-five minutes," he said cheerfully.

My cries were still ringing in Bill's ears when Dr. Yu approached him with arm outstretched in greeting. To Bill, that gesture only meant "You're next!" He jumped up and declared that his toe was absolutely fine.

Later I saw the holes burned in Bill's jacket when a cigarette dropped unnoticed from his shaking hand. He hadn't even smelled the burning cloth.

Dr. Yu was still laughing when he came to remove the needles at the end of my treatment. "You have performed a miracle cure. Your screams have cured your husband's toe."

By nighttime I had discounted the pain of the acupuncture and the bloated foot began to feel as if it did belong to me. The weird swelling was receding and as it did, some warmth stole down to the frozen toes. In the morning I could actually feel the bones of my right foot and I was so happy that I called Dr. Yu immediately.

Two days after the acupuncture the swelling had almost entirely disappeared, but I became conscious of a strange new sensation of numbness that began in the right foot but soon crept upward until both my legs and buttocks were affected. There was no pain, no warning, and suddenly no feeling—sitting in the bath, I suddenly could not feel the bottom of the tub. I had to watch my legs moving to be sure that I was getting out of the water. I had to look in the mirror to see if I were dry! I called Dr. Yu at once. He listened and answered reassuringly, "Don't worry, it will go away."

But it didn't go away. The numbness persisted, intensified. We were due to go to the country for the long Memorial Day weekend and Bill was so alarmed by the idea of my condition worsening when we were far from the doctor that he ran down the block to Dr. Yu's office to see if there might be anything that could be done for me.

Again, the doctor was unalarmed, reassuring. "It will go away," he told Bill calmly.

The weekend was quiet but we were so uneasy that we came back to town early.

The next day a terrible, twisting pain attacked my midriff, burning like high-voltage shock. It didn't pass, it didn't lessen, it shrieked and jangled inside my ribs until I gasped over the phone to Dr. Yu, "I think this pain will drive me mad!"

His voice was soothing, sympathetic. "It sounds like a flare-up of the intercostal nerves. Try to get as much rest as you can. It will go away."

I couldn't even sit in one place, I couldn't do anything but hobble around the room on my wooden legs, fighting the pain with movement. I called Dr. Stock. He was sympathetic too. "Come to my office tomorrow," he said.

By the next day that was impossible. I was no longer moving around: the slightest quiver of motion made the pain worse. We cancelled the appoin ment with Dr. Stock, turned back to Dr. Yu only a block away. Again, Bill ran down to his office and told him that he must think of someting to do for me.

And, again, the doctor said that there was nothing to do. It would go away.

Bill called Dr. Stock for another appointment, but I had to cancel again because I was in such agony. I couldn't crawl to see the doctor. I wondered why he didn't suggest coming to see me. The incredible fact was that I was unable to communicate the intensity of my pain; the glass wall was in place: my doctors couldn't hear me. Neither man suggested a pain-killer. I had the conviction that I would shoot myself if the pain did not soon abate.

It took me six pain-wracked days to collect myself enough to see Dr. Stock in his office. I had lost six pounds: barely eaten, could not remember sleeping. I heard Dr. Stock say, after he had finished his examination: "I could send you to the Neurological Institute at the Medical Center but that would be overreacting. After all, I have the same tools here."

I nodded numbly.

"Watch the nerves," added Dr. Stock suddenly. "When they go, they go fast."

What was I to watch for? I wondered if he meant that I was about to have a nervous breakdown. I felt I would if the pain was not soon relieved. Just to exist, to endure the immediate moments, I needed sleep and relief from pain. If I hadn't been a cancer patient and had appeared in his office after six days of such pain, I am sure Dr. Stock would have ordered an ambulance immediately. But invariably a cancer patient's doctor wears "cancer blinders"; the patient's other ailments are seen as insignificant by comparison and treated perfunctorily.

I left his office without anything to alleviate my pain.

We had stumbled back to our apartment to face another sleepless night, when the telephone rang.

The caller was an old friend, a European doctor who was visiting New York. Bill seized the phone. "Come over at once; Joie needs you!"

She was there in twenty minutes. I could judge my appearance by the look in her eyes. "My God, Joie, call your doctor!"

"I have just come from my doctor." I was half sobbing as I told her the story.

She didn't stop to sympathize. "Call him. Tell him you must have a prescription for pain and sleeping pills. You cannot go on like this."

I called Dr. Stock and repeated her message. He called a druggist and arranged for medication over the phone. It was as simple as that.

That night I slept a dull, dazed sleep, waking automatically at four-hour intervals for fresh pills. I slept on and off through the next day and wakened with an appetite. When I slept again, it was a natural, luxurious nap. The numbness still persisted in my legs but was no worse and the wracking pain in my midriff had leached away to a manageable discomfort. The world looked so much sweeter to me that I rose like Lazarus and announced that we could go to the country after all. I even called both doctors to report my improvement.

On Sunday I was free from pain. After a lovely, leisurely morning, I walked into my bedroom for a midday nap. When I awoke, I raised my head—and could go no further. At first I thought the numbness in my hips and legs had returned full strength, but slowly I discovered that I could not move my hips and legs at all. They lay on the bed, stone-rigid, without feeling. Above my waist I was capable of movement; below it, nothing.

I thought it was a progression of the numbness, a temporary inability to move. My mind rushed to cling to that position: I thought of Dr. Yu's calm assurances that "it will go away." Surely he had enough experience to back that certainty, surely this new development had a remedy. Wait. Lie still. Feeling and mobility may flow in again. Don't panic, don't act on panic yet, don't call out to Bill.

It was in this same bedroom, a little more than one year ago, that I had told Bill that I could not see with my left eye. I had awakened from sleep then, too, and imagined a temporary blindness. But I mustn't make parallels, must not interpret fate; this numbness did not strike at me suddenly like the eye, it's been gradual, not a thunderclap. There must be a therapy for it.

I heard Bill outside the bedroom window, working in the garden. Gently, I tried out my voice.

"Bill? Come into the bedroom. I want to tell you something."

I heard him digging: imagined his hands full of seedlings. "Come out to the garden, love. Tell me here."

I froze in terror. I would not be walking out into the garden! He would have to come in to me; and I would unveil this newest horror. How could Bill endure still another unfolding terror?

I needn't have been so cautious for Bill's sake. He reacted as I had, refusing to accept the idea of paralysis, convinced that this was a progression of my problem and one that would respond to drugs. Hadn't the searing pain in my midriff disappeared with medicine? I faltered, wondering if that was only because the bonfire of my nerve endings had finally burned out. But Bill would not let me wonder. He said, "Suppose I stand you on your feet? Then you can try to stand alone."

But it didn't work. From the waist down not a muscle moved.

First we called Dr. Stock. He was out of town, would be back on Monday. There seemed little point in discussing what had happened with the doctor who was covering his calls, even less point to driving in to Columbia Presbyterian when most of its doctors were absent. "Most of them are probably right out here in the Hamptons," Bill muttered. No, we'd use the hours between then and the next morning to make practical arrangements.

In rapid succession, Bill called our housekeeper at her home, then a handyman and then Dr. Merle, the local general practitioner who'd been so helpful during my eye crisis. Then Bill retreated to a storage room and returned dragging one of our prize antique-shop trophies, a Hitchcock armchair with a chaise seat originally designed to house a chamber pot.

"You'll need a portable bathroom, won't you?" Then he brought in a kitty litter pan. He tried to fit it into the hinged compartment under the chair but it was slightly too wide.

"I thought so," Bill nodded. "The handyman will shave these sides down."

So there was my throne. My husband had an answer for everything. And he had thoughtfully provided me with another set of problems to occupy my mind; I would have to direct the housekeeper to pack for me, make decisions on what I needed in the hospital for however long I had to stay there.

Dr. Merle arrived more in the role of friend than physician. But he did examine me for all of the vital signs and kept a sharp professional eye on me throughout the day, watching, I know now, for signs of shock or breathing difficulties. But there was nothing. No fingers of numbness crept toward my chest—and I think I was past the idea of shock. I could not hope or fear the uncertain events of the future; I could only wait, exist until Monday morning.

Monday began in confusion. Bill wanted to drive me in to the hospital himself but Dr. Merle suggested that an ambulance could cut through the Monday expressway jam and shorten the journey. So we ordered the ambulance, but it was away on an out-of-town emergency. Bill picked me up and carried me into the back seat of our car; cradled me in pillows and fastened me in place. We would go directly to Columbia Presbyterian; Dr. Stock had said that he'd be waiting for us with a neurosurgeon. I could let my mind play with the possibility of surgery . . . I had to believe that they would do something at the hospital to give me the use of my legs. But if my inability to move was due to something pressing on my spine, something that must be excised, what could it be but another tumor? And if it was, what had been the use of taking all the recent tests I had had to prove myself free from cancer?

At the hospital the neurosurgeon immediately confirmed my apprehension by dismissing the painful acupuncture as a possible trigger for the disaster and concentrating instead on inevitability of a tumor on my spine. He felt sure it was there, sure he could get it. But hours were precious, deterioration swift, we must not wait. A special scan called a milogram would pinpoint the tumor's location on my spine and surgery could follow immediately. We had only to sign the release.

Only three months ago I had been declared free of detectable cancer in Germany. And after that I was examined here in this hospital when my wooden foot began its final antics. Of course they had not looked at the spine for cancer during that examination, just as they had not looked behind my eyes the year before or into my right lung to detect the tumor found in Germany. No, the word "detectable" suggests an efficiency that does not exist! If this was still another cancerous tumor, then cancer was playing hopscotch through my body well ahead of all the doctors' efforts at "detection." In the depth of my mind another, lower, depth opened, threatening to devour me. There was no bottom to futility, no trust in assurances served up by a science that has not found a cancer cure. The doctor told me that surgery could relieve the paralysis, but beyond that, there could be no promises or guarantees. Still, hope is an irrepressible instinct. I signed the release and we waited for the milogram that would tell the story.

We waited for two hours: I, lying on a stretcher; Bill and the neurosurgeon, Dr. Edgar Housepian, standing beside me in the sub-basement corridor outside the milogram room. The milogram machine was in use for other emergencies. The hospital technicians were on a work slowdown preceding a strike, so everything was slowed down. An operating room was being made available. Bill had time to call Dick and Stephanie in Puerto Rico, Dick's plane had the time to complete half its journey to New York, the surgeon had more time than he wanted to calculate and recalculate my chances. Suddenly he pulled us out of the purgatory of waiting by deciding to operate without the milogram. It would be more difficult but his judgment found it imperative to wait no longer.

I began to try to add the days, estimate the time I had spent in hospitals waiting for surgery, treatment or recovery in the past two years. It occupied me on the ride to the operating room. Bill walked close beside me, holding my hand, pressing my fingers lightly. I was retreating slowly from the lights and sound and noise when the stretcher stopped. Just stopped. Bill leaned close and whispered, "The technician from the milogram room has just come down. It's free now. The surgeon wants to go there first."

Mercifully he did. After a thorough, one-hour scan with the milogram machine there was no evidence of a tumor on my spine, none whatsoever. Cancer had not reached that site. Dr. Housepian was a very honorable man; he shared his relief and confusion with us openly. He told us that I had been minutes away from unnecessary surgery on the spine! No cancerous tumor was causing my paralysis; no tumor was there. I wondered how long it would be until, or if, we would find the answer and I could move and walk again.

I lay in a semi-private Intensive Care ward, here because the threat of a hospital strike three weeks away had crowded patients into Harkness like so many vegetables in a bin. Even though Dr. Stock was a member of the hospital's Board of Directors, he had not been able to arrange for the private room the neurologist insisted was necessary. To my left a dying old woman was receiving the last rites in Hungarian from her bedside priest. Beyond her lay a woman still comatose from lung cancer surgery earlier in the day. Another woman, more fully recovered, kept complaining loudly and calling for the nurse. She almost succeeded in drowning out the "Ba, ba, ba!" of a senile patient who sat bolt upright in her bed nodding and bleating continuously. Not twelve feet away from me, through an open doorway, I could see the busy nurses' station, and hear it too: phones frantically jangling, nurses pounding back and forth on errands, lights flashing emergency. The old woman's hoarse voice grew louder, the better to be heard by her approaching God, the old lady's bleat rose triumphantly as antiphon—yet my neurologist's advice upon entering my case was, "What you need, above anything else, is absolute tranquility and rest."

After two days of poking and flexing my inert legs the neurologist thought that he had discovered my problem: radiation burns on the spinal column. He told Bill and Dick and me that if he was correct in this diagnosis it meant that I would never regain the use of my legs. We were turned into a tableau as rigid as my frozen legs as we heard this latest grave sentence pronounced, had this latest bit broken off our lives.

I was not in pain. I would have welcomed pain below my waist but there was no stir of feeling in the dead weight of hips and legs. A sudden rush of motion images flickered through my mind. I remembered beating the boys at ice skating on a pine-rimmed pond, I remembered each separate sensation of running on the beach with Bill, the air gliding down my body, the wind streaming through my hair, the ball of my foot just skimming the sand. There was no escape from these images of lightness and release. If I had not been so active, it might be easier to learn passivity, learn to accept being lifted, bundled, carried, wheeled, bathed, forever "done unto," forever an object, forever a lumpen weight. What would happen to the free design for living that Bill and I had created? What would happen to the man and woman who loved each other? Sleep was barely possible in the four days and nights I spent in the Intensive Care ward; I had plenty of time to torture myself with the future. I thought of all the ways in which I would now be a burden to the ones I loved. Could they survive my transmutation to a lumpen thing?

After four days and nights had passed, two nurses and an orderly came to transfer me to a private room. I weighed one hundred and ten pounds; it took three of them to fight the drag of absolute dead weight and maneuver me onto the stretcher. One of the nurses told me that I would learn to do transfers for myself. I didn't believe her, didn't think the leaden lump would even learn to do anything that produced motion, but I pushed and pulled with my arms obediently as if I had something real to accomplish.

Dr. Stock had finally succeeded in having me installed in a lovely room with a river view. I had the private nurses I needed, nurses prohibited by hospital rule in Intensive Care, and I had a team of specialists cooperating on my case: one neurologist, two physical therapists, one physical doctor, Dr. Stock, an oncologist, and a new arrival, the urologist—urgently needed because my bladder was nonfunctioning and I was being catheterized several times a day. At times the traffic in my room grew chaotic. Bill, in spite of his efforts to arrive at a time when I was alone, would spend hours in the waiting room while I was being poked, prodded, medicated and discussed by several doctors who had converged on my room at the same time. They got in each other's way. After a particularly bad stack-up one afternoon, I insisted that each doctor and therapist give me a particular time when he would visit. The doctors accepted the idea but the therapists balked until I made a chart showing the flow of traffic and insisted that they agree on a schedule. I had to do it because they were taking away the one thing I desperately needed: my time with Bill.

Bill and I waited a week before the doctors would give any more definite opinions. Luckily, Dick had been able to stay with Bill all that time before he flew back to Puerto Rico and his wife and the new son he had barely seen. He'd been summoned to my bedside for yet another crisis on the same day that Stephanie came home from the hospital with the baby. But his company was providential for Bill, essential to me. Dick was the balance wheel that kept us from flying to pieces while we waited. And there was a welcome touch of normalcy in the thought that I was now a grandmother: that there would be baby pictures in the mail. I needed every thread to tie myself to life.

When the doctors finally arrived at their conclusions about my situation they were quite divided in their opinions. But there was consensus on the origin of my paralysis: a condition called mylopathy. Because of overradiation, the nerve centers in my spinal cord crucial to motion in the lower half of my body had gradually weakened and then "burned out." The numbness in my right foot, existing for months, might have been a symptom of mylopathy. Was that why the acupuncture had been so painful, or had the acupuncture itself triggered the burn-out of nerves? Everyone wanted to avoid answering my question because no one could be sure; it was terra incognita.

Dr. Stock said, "They overradiated you in Germany."

"Germany? Why Germany? I had very little radiation there. But I had a great deal of deep radiation right here in this hospital."

It was all useless, after the fact. We could easily have sunk to accusing, demanding, contradicting, exposing raw resentments—but I'd still be flat on my back. There was no use feeling bitterness. I didn't want to begin a ritual of blame, I only wanted a medical miracle.

For a time, my miracle didn't seem out of reach. The original opinion of the hospital's top neurologist, Dr. Daniel Sciarra, had been that I would never have the use of my legs again. After three days he reversed himself. He saw hopeful indications in my response to medication and exercise. With practice, I could move my feet in circles, I could wiggle my toes back and forth—a wondrous pleasure. After more sessions with the therapists I was even able to lift my legs from the bed just a little so that Dr. Sciarra could see "air space" between the bed and the legs. It was spectacular progress in terms of reflex action and resurfacing sensation in my legs and feet. For a while I was so happy with it that I managed not to think of my frozen bladder. In spite of the urologist's arsenal of drugs to restore the bladder's function, I still needed the catheter every four hours around the clock.

I had nurses around the clock and they were busy with the catheterizations, the medicines, the chart, the reports to the doctors and the personal attention to the large, stiff wooden doll in their care who could bend at the elbows but not at the knees. My room was banked with all the flowers Bill could bring in from our garden. My hospital menu was supplemented with delicacies. We were still Hans and Fritz because we couldn't get it through our heads that this time we might be beaten. Ours were feasts of optimism: the cold lobsters perfectly packed in ice that Bill brought one Sunday afternoon clearly said we'd overcome, the garden-fresh sorrel soup revived memories of Georgetown Hospital and our brave last supper with Dick and Stephanie before the bad dream became reality. And when, after the third week, the neurologist decided that I could sit up in a wheelchair wearing a corset reinforced with steel stays, Hans and Fritz seized on this sign of progress and swung happily into the search for a steel-boned corset, size eight.

But a size eight steel-stayed corset was a contradiction in terms, apparently, an anomaly not to be found in a retail shop or at the wholesale level or through the manufacturers Bill knew. Even the stores that sell trusses and crutches and wheelchairs disappointed us. We were baffled until the day that Bill's usual supply of parking spaces around the hospital failed him and he was forced to look for a spot on Broadway, blocks away. There in a seedy neighborhood, with stores surviving from a more prosperous time, was exactly the kind of corset emporium that existed decades ago. It was the sort of place that no longer existed in the more fashionable areas downtown, but here there was still a need, because women still showed and suffered the effects on the body from too many childbirths, outsize proportions because ''a woman should have something on her bones,'' or presurgical attempts to correct nature's inequities. A steel-boned size eight corset would not be laughed at here! Bill stepped inside to speak with the owner, and a half-hour later the good man was taking my measurements in the hospital and laying out samples of stays for the decisions of the neurologist and physical doctor.

The neurologist and the physical doctor had different ideas about my future. The physical doctor, who supervised my therapists, felt that I was doing well enough to be sent home in a wheelchair in ten days and expect to eventually graduate to a walker, while the neurologist told me that the walker was unlikely because my spine would never be strong enough. The first news filled us with hope—even a geriatric shuffle inside a walker was mobility—but the second dashed that spark. I had to take into account that the physical doctor had been proven overoptimistic—he was Dr. Yu, who had assured me not to worry because "It will go away."

Doctors from my past came by to view me in my present complication. I suppose I was a curiosity because I was still alive. I think I said so to Dr. Sciarra and he laughed. He was Olympian but warm and involved. He did not begrudge explanations. He positively lectured me; coaxing, cajoling and prying progress from my reluctant legs. His warm brown eyes could grow suspiciously moist. And he was not afraid to reverse his professional opinion when new evidence appeared; he had gone from the dictum that I would never move my legs again to the notion that I might stand with crutches someday. But time would have to make that decision. Clearly, there was not much reason to extend my stay in the hospital. Dr. Sciarra saw my main problem as adjustment and wanted earnestly to smooth my way in the world outside.

"You should spend four months at the Rusk Institute," he told me in one conversation. "Go there from here. They can do a lot for you in therapy and they can show you how to deal with your new situation."

"Are you saying that I should go there to learn how to be a cripple?"

"Well, how do you plan to learn?"

"I don't. I don't plan to think of myself in any different way than I do now."

"But you'll have to. You'll have to govern your life, hold everything together."

I smiled. Fortunately, I already knew how to do that.

"I don't want to learn to function as a cripple. I'm going to try to continue to be myself, just robbed of mobility now."

"Rusk Institute could still help."

"Doctor Sciarra, if you saw me like this as the result of an accident, I'd go immediately to Rusk Institute for rehabilitation. But I am a patient with a history of metastasized cancer. Wouldn't I be foolish to squander four months of my precious time away from the people and the things I love? I want to spend every moment with them."

He understood so well that his next words were, "When do you want to leave the hospital?"

"When do you think I should?"

He considered it. "You can plan on leaving within the next five days. Of course there will be a few problems, a few things you must learn how to do before you leave."

That was a valiant understatement. I was still practicing the transfer maneuver in and out of my wheelchair and there was still the obstacle of the catheterization needed three times a day. But my doctors decided in conference with the urologist that I should learn to catheterize myself.

I protested, "I can't do it!"

Dr. Stock's logic finally stopped my objections. By my own words, I did not intend to function as a cripple. Bill and I would probably travel, we would certainly be in the country each weekend, and unless we were prepared to assume the permanent burden of living and traveling with a nurse, I must learn to use the catheter. And Bill should learn as well.

"Not Bill," I said. "I would like to spare him *something*." But I was wrong to think that I could.

My first attempt at using the catheter was rather like committing self-surgery as I peered into a mirror and tried to follow the nurse's instructions. There was a lot of necessary equipment: a standup mirror, the metal catheter, which must be sterile in the towel in which it was autoclaved, a washbasin, a flashlight, sterile cotton, sterile gloves, sterile jelly and pillows to prop under the legs, frog-fashion, so that the process could begin.

Step by step, I committed these instructions to memory. Spread the vulva with the left hand. Pick up the metal catheter with the right hand, making sure that it touches nothing that would break the sterile condition. Locate the miatus, a small opening above the vagina. Notice that the catheter is curved at the point of insertion and must be inserted first with a dipping motion and then with an instant lift as soon as it passes through the opening of the miatus. Push the catheter into the bladder and hold it there until voiding is complete. The sterile condition must not be broken anywhere during the process. If it happens, the equipment must be resterilized and the catheterization begun again. These precautions are taken because contamination is an ever-present problem and everything must be done to avoid the development of bladder infections.

Mercifully, the sight in my right eye had grown keener through increased use and I had long since learned to compensate for the loss of full perspective. And mercifully too, the metal catheter was faster than the plastic model the nurses had been using on me. I found the miatus on my second try. With each success, I felt a small pride. This I could do; I would be independent here.

A great deal of equipment would be needed now for the simplest daily living. I would not go home without the wheelchair, commodes, a sterilizer, the catheterization equipment and the plastic slide boards needed to transfer from chair to bed, bed to chair. I called this "my safari" and on the day of discharge from the hospital I expected to leave by amublance while my equipment followed in another car.

Bill vetoed that. "I'll pack the equipment in our car," he said. "And no ambulance. I got her here, I'll get her home."

We had hired a practical nurse and she was waiting at our country place. We'd be there for the rest of the summer; everything was arranged there for my comfort. But Bill and I had another immediate idea which we didn't mention to the doctors until the day prior to leaving. They reacted as we'd known they would:

"Why do you want to stay overnight in the city?"

"You'll have to unpack everything for just one night. It will be monumental trouble."

"The nurse is in the country. How will you manage?"

Frankly, that was what we wanted to find out. Of course there were things in our city apartment that I wanted to take to the country, but there was an emotional reason, too. It would be the first time we'd confront the new life together and the last time alone, without other people's helping hands, for months to come. "Let's touch base," I said. "Let's touch base and see how it's going to be."

We stayed overnight and took our traumas as they landed on us. The transfer from the wheelchair to the bed was ghastly; still we managed to drag my leaden body across the slide board without accident. We got through three catheterizations without a nurse, and Bill charted the schedule of all my medications and treatments so that there could be no possible mistake. This overnight coping, this practice run was necessary to our future. Something could be salvaged of the old days, we could try to live with some of the same old spirit that colored our lives with zest and anticipation. The only other choice was complete resignation. Even though the odds were heavily against us, we decided to try to live our lives completely, to the full extent of our now limited capacity.

## CHAPTER XVI

# Our Life Today

My first weeks at home as a paraplegic were in some ways like the time, seemingly ages ago, when I had first found out that I had cancer. I felt the same disbelief: the absolute impossibility of understanding that my life had been wrenched into a terrible new shape, and that I was unable to do anything about it. I heard the same echoing of slamming doors as possibilities closed themselves to me forever. And I sank into the same empty shock and grief at the prospect of trying to find some semblance of a normal life within the very limited capabilities of the body which I had left.

Bill still clung to hope, and devised theories and dreams about when and how I'd walk again. I came to believe the doctors' diagnosis that the radiation therapy which had burned out my tumors had also burned out the nerves in my spinal column, and that the paralysis was irreversible. It seemed a vicious irony to have achieved such a prolonged remission of cancer and then to be chained to the radius I could navigate in a wheelchair, my legs burnt offerings which had gained me life.

At first I cursed the bargain that had bought my life at such a price, for my immobility was a dehumanizing process: I had to

be bathed, drained of urine three times a day and hauled and
lifted about like a sack. The helplessness led first to despondency, then to shame and frustration at my inability to do even
ridiculously simple things for myself. I could not accept myself
as passive object once again. Especially since this time it was to
be for life.

I had a lot of time for reflection and often wondered if there
might have been an alternative to the cancer assembly line
which bore me so swiftly through surgery, radiation and
chemotherapy. Perhaps if I had known about the phenomenon
of spontaneous remission of cancer *prior* to undergoing
surgery, I might have decided against taking the conventional
cancer therapy entirely. I might have chosen to take my chances
in a different sort of way. I might even have survived—to this
day—whole and unmutilated, standing on my own two feet.
But it is impossible to tell whether success, it if comes at all,
comes from standard treatment or from still un-understood
causes in the awesome enterprise of fighting cancer. Each
cancer case is different. Some victims benefit from treatment
and lengthen their lives. Others are cured by the baffling spontaneous remissions which do occur.

Bill guessed at the doubts that haunted me and he made me
understand what we had to do: find the strength and spirit to spit
in the eye of fate once more and keep on living. He gallantly
went about living our life as if I were not a burden. In the fall we
began going back and forth from city to country each week
having friends and family and business associates by for lunch
or dinner, very much as we had eons ago, when I was a vigorous
pillar of health. Bill now did all of the preparation for those
occasions, did all of the work in the garden, did everything to
keep our lives running, and did it while carrying me around or
pushing me from place to place in a wheelchair.

It did not happen at once, but slowly, by clinging determinedly to the fragments of the life we used to have, by forgetting

what can't be replaced and turning away from the impossible, we are refashioning a life that is still in our image. We get along without the 24-hour nurses. We liked more privacy. A nurse comes every morning now and is gone by noon. I am still Bill's partner and planner via the phone. We entertain, we have guests. We work, perhaps with even greater determination than before. We go out around town, though our trips are now limited to places that don't present serious problems for a wheelchair.

This is not life as we once lived it. But we have found that we can endure more than I had thought possible in the beginning. Nine months have passed since half of my body has died. I range backward through my memories and forward into hope; it balances the inertia of the present. For a time my mind was as leaden as my legs, now I stir again, now I spend time in the future, thinking of how it will be when I gather my energies against this last, latest obstacle to living. I cannot live in despair. Some of what we formerly enjoyed is still present; a little color, a little zest, much stubborn curiosity.

We find, Bill and I, that our life together still offers many profound satisfactions. And we find, after all we've been through that, more than ever before, we can share whatever joy and contentment come to us.

# An Afternote

## by Richard Harrison

       Shortly after she completed this book, Joie McGrail suffered a recurrence of lung cancer and died.

When my mother first confronted cancer she set three goals for herself: to maintain her spirit, to do everything possible to prolong her life, and to really enjoy as much as possible the extra time she could win for herself through determination. She achieved all of her goals.

Joie looked cancer in the eye and didn't flinch. She managed to stretch a post-operative life expectancy of six months to three years. And she filled those years with a richness of experience, happiness and enjoyment.

In those three years Joie and Bill, who had always had an extraordinarily close relationship, grew nearer and more loving every day. They enjoyed their country cottage and continued their constant round of changes and improvements. More cats were found and adopted, more antiques were squeezed into already crammed rooms. Her first grandchildren were born, and Joie met them and began to experience a new joy, the thrill of being a grandmother.

And in the years she gained Joie wrote this book, a project

which was very important to her. She felt that her experiences with cancer, and her responses to the terrible challenges which the disease presents might help other victims question their methods of treatment and find means of coping with the disease or even winning the battle. She felt that she herself had faced the challenge and been victorious and she was right. She had kept her spirit, prolonged her life and truly enjoyed the extra time she had won for herself.

It was a triumph of will and love, bravery and sharing. Her strong, joyful spirit overcame the fear and suffering of a dreaded disease.